Contents

USING
CHILD PSYCHIATRY

Derek Steinberg trained in medicine at the London
Hospital Medical College and in psychiatry at the
Maudsley and Bethlem Royal Hospitals, the
National Hospital for Nervous Diseases, the
Tavistock Clinic and the Park Hospital for Children
in Oxford. He was appointed consultant psy-
chiatrist at the Regional Adolescent Unit, Long
Grove Hospital, in 1973, and to the Maudsley
Hospital in 1975, where he is currently consultant
psychiatrist to the Department of Child and Ado-
lescent Psychiatry and in charge of the Adolescent
Unit at Bethlem Royal Hospital.

TEACH YOURSELF BOOKS

To
Anna, Catherine and Gill
for their forbearance with my first

USING CHILD PSYCHIATRY

The Functions and Operations of a Specialty

Derek Steinberg

Consultant psychiatrist, Department of Child and Adolescent Psychiatry, The Maudsley Hospital, and the Adolescent Unit, Bethlem Royal Hospital

Illustrated by Vanessa Pancheri

TEACH YOURSELF BOOKS

Hodder and Stoughton

First printed 1981

Copyright © 1981
Derek Steinberg

British Library Cataloguing in Publication Data

Steinberg, Derek
Using child psychiatry
1. Child psychiatry
I. Title
618.92'89   RJ499

ISBN 0 340 26835 2

Printed and bound in Great Britain
for Hodder and Stoughton paperbacks, a division of
Hodder and Stoughton Ltd, Mill Road, Dunton Green,
Sevenoaks, Kent (Editorial Office: 47 Bedford Square,
London, WC1B 3DP) by Richard Clay
(The Chaucer Press) Ltd, Bungay, Suffolk
Photoset by Rowland Phototypesetting Ltd,
Bury St Edmunds, Suffolk

He who would do good to another must do it in
Minute Particulars
General Good is the plea of the scoundrel, hypocrite and
flatterer;
For Art and Science cannot exist but in minutely
organised particulars

William Blake

Preface:
A Guide to the Book

This book is not another short account of child psychiatry for non-psychiatrists. There are several good short guides already, and they appear in the reading list (p. 191). Rather, it is an attempt to describe how child and adolescent psychiatry fits into the very wide range of overlapping services the adult world provides for children. This requires some description of child development and child psychiatry, but this is kept to the minimum necessary to describe what child psychiatrists and their colleagues are like, and how they think and work. It also means dipping into philosophy and semantics and professional politics here and there, because there is a good deal of muddle and disorder in the child-care field; so the book is also something of a balancing act between how things are and how, at least in the writer's view, they ought to be.

The book is planned to be a guide to a perplexing and multifarious subject, but it is not a reference handbook; it is not planned to be dipped into for an account of the treatment of conduct disorders or the addresses of psychiatric clinics. It is designed to be read through reasonably quickly and to convey in broad outline what the large numbers of people in child psychiatry and related fields are up to: the lines along which child psychiatrists think and the sort of action they take; and a recurring theme of the book is the question: what is child psy-

chiatry for? what can it do that other professionals, or
other people for that matter, cannot? This is an uncomfortable question, but a few steps towards answering it
will be ultimately helpful for child psychiatry as much as
for everybody else. There are other recurring themes
too, and to this extent there is some deliberate repetition
and elaboration of certain points made, which are looked
at more than once from different angles: for example
what an angry and unhappy child may be like in a
children's home, how the child's problems may be
categorised diagnostically and, later on, how professional
workers might usefully get together to help the boy or
girl and, better still, prevent psychiatric crises in the
first place.

I hope the book will be comprehensible to any interested adult, but it is written with professional workers
in mind. I have tended to refer in the text to *clinical
workers*, meaning child psychiatrists and those working
directly with them, such as clinic and hospital social
workers and psychologists, and *other professional
workers*, meaning for example education welfare officers,
'field' social workers, educational psychologists and
teachers, and it is these two broad groups of professionals
the book is for. So turbulent is the field that even to
mention this in the Preface touches immediately on
controversy: for example social workers and educational
psychologists are often far from comfortably established
in clinical teams. If they are firmly based in the team,
who should be in charge, psychiatrist, social worker or
psychologist? If it depends on what the team is trying to
do, is that always clear? What sort of response is needed
when a frightened child goes wild? Staff counselling?
An injection? Radical social reform? Psychotherapy? As
the book moves from vantage point to vantage point to
look at problems from different points of view, there is
one thread for the reader to hold on to: adults must work
together with reasonable competence and mutual confidence if we are to help children, and particularly

children in trouble. By and large we don't, and this needs looking at, even if it will lead to arguments.

Two points about the strategy of the book. First, although for the most part I have emphasised the problems that occur in this field of work, large numbers of boys and girls are being well looked after, or competently treated if treatment is what they need, by social service departments, special schools and child psychiatric clinics up and down the country. The people I have met and worked with in all the various professions concerned have included very many who have struck me as being among the most hard-working and conscientious in any industry, and more genuinely concerned with their responsibilities than most. Nor is it easy work. People in the child care field are quite often told, sometimes by the same people and in the same breath, that their work is somehow a cushy number and yet at the same time that it must be really awful and how on earth do they put up with it. In fact it can be extraordinarily demanding work, if done properly, and among the easiest in which to cut corners. I have tended not to dwell on good work, or procedures that go smoothly, but there is a great deal of good work and smooth procedure.

Second, the book has a sequence. It begins with a survey of the field and an emergency in a children's home to illustrate a number of central issues, and introduces an approach to help the reader conceptualise needs and problems on the one hand and resources and solutions on the other. In the following chapters needs and problems are elaborated by chapters outlining child development and disorder, and in particular disorder as conceptualised by psychiatrists; and resources by a chapter on treatment, again from the psychiatric point of view. The quite different styles of response to children's problems, psychiatric and otherwise, are put into an historical context by a brief account of how different services for children have developed. The closing chapters are about how professional workers need to get together in children's interests, and the sort of things that can make this difficult. The book ends with some thoughts about the future of child psychiatry within the broader perspectives of child care and education.

The book has a number of roots, and I would like to acknowledge them. It has partly grown out of seminars I have taken over the years at the University of Surrey's sociology department, and has been prompted and I hope benefited by much talking through of the issues that follow by post-graduates from many different professions and with very different points of view. I am similarly grateful to my colleagues at the Adolescent Unit, Bethlem Royal Hospital, from whom I continue to learn, to Jean Winship, the Unit's secretary, who typed the many successive drafts, and to my wife, Gill, for her forbearance during the book's gestation, and for preparing the index.

Finally, the examples described in the book are deliberately jumbled so that particular children's homes, departments and people cannot be identified by the facts given. Any suspicion of familiarity is because the examples, disputes and eccentricities described are all common ones: matters which the newcomer to the field may regard as quite extraordinary soon turn out to be quite routine.

Derek Steinberg
Bethlem Royal Hospital, 1981

I

Introduction:
The Field Surveyed

A curious business is the phenomenon of child psychiatry. In every age large numbers of adults have found children difficult to understand and manage except when, as a matter of common sense, handling them ruthlessly and sometimes brutally. In this century 'common sense' is treated more guardedly – in many industrialised communities there is no common consensus – and a sense of uncertainty, and an ambivalent but persisting faith in the specialist, has resulted in large numbers of people being prepared to turn for advice about children to the expert in madness.

In the rest of the animal world parenthood is an all-or-none affair. At first infants are looked after very thoroughly; then they fend for themselves, and the adults return to the literally vital business that underwrites further reproduction: individual and group survival.

The human race is different. Human children take years to become self-sufficient in even the most elementary way, and as the world has become more sophisticated (a splendid word that means among other things elaborate, complicated, fallacious, misleading) children now take some eighteen to twenty-five years to become self-supporting adults, during which time their parents are engaged in developing their own lives further, a process which in some cases includes, in a sense, a prolonged adolescence and the search for a philosophy of living as well as the prolonged pursuit of career, mortgage etc. This is not to denigrate such pursuits. The adult world now has some very real uncertainties to cope with. The rights and wrongs of ambitions and behaviour are controversial. Matters about which there was once solid clarity – like thrift, discipline, education, patriotism, the law – now polarise people. If you don't like your husband, wife, child, parents, it is no longer taken for granted that you have to learn to live with them. You can change your name, face, sex, for that matter. Technical advances have made possible the survival of handicapped children who would have died, provided tidy ways of dealing with conception, brought in new forms of toxicity affecting development, and encouraged the notion, vague and compelling, that there are, or ought to be, ways of correcting anything uncomfortable or unusual. Nor is this an entirely empty promise, and that makes it even more difficult. Adults – parents – are no longer sure where they stand, nor what they have to put up with.

A lot is expected of children too. It is not merely a matter of simply supporting, say, a retarded child and his parents when special education and treatment might help too. Social possibilities are vast, and no one is going to leave a bunch of children going fishing, lunching off pinched apples and helping the local shopkeepers any more when they ought to be in school. There are big important things to get on with and learn; there really are, and a child needs not only a reasonably stable home, but a reasonably stable mood and ability to concentrate, reasonably predictable and conforming social behaviours, and a reasonable level of intelligence to cope with it all. If he falls behind educationally or because of some variation in attitude or mood, there are ways of helping him get right again.

One might think that the categories of help needed by children in difficulties were relatively few. In fact children's problems have led to a most extraordinary proliferation of experts, services and theories. These continue to expand in a most profligate way, budding off new units and new areas of expertise with a fecundity limited more by lack of funds than because adequate thought and study has demonstrated what is or isn't needed. If the local child psychiatric clinic has a three-month waiting list, then appoint another psychiatrist! The adolescent unit is always full up; submit plans for a new one! Or (for there are lots of forward looking people in the field) start a day hospital, or a family therapy clinic, or a psychodrama centre.

In a hypothetical march-past in a prosperous welfare state of the future, who might go swinging past the podium on Child Care Day? Social workers in serried ranks, area banners and department emblems flying; then a group of developmental assessment specialists accompanied by clinical and research workers in paed-iatrics, then a detachment of specialist lawyers and representatives of twenty or thirty ginger groups, in-cluding some MPs. Then a formation of borstal staff and special hospital personnel (adolescent division) followed by cohorts of academic sociologists, psychologists and educationalists, with a squad of action and experiential therapists moving briskly up behind. There follows, on a succession of lorries, demonstrations representing secure units, behaviour therapy units, junior prisons and the short, sharp shock, therapeutic communities and special schools, intermediate treatment units, day attendance centres, school counsellors, educational therapists, and drug rehabilitation communities. A float passes representing different styles of children's remand, assessment and emergency reception centres, and then the brass band of the child and adolescent psychiatrists appears. In the distance we see a column of probation officers moving forward swiftly like Ghurkas, and behind them come remedial teachers, police officers (juvenile bureaux), health visitors, Area and District community physicians (Child Health and Mental Health), school medical officers, and then the massed bands of the clinical psychologists, clashing inharmoniously with those of the educational psychologists, with child psychologists coming up too. Behind them, just turning the corner, comes a unit of child psychotherapists. Marking time around the corner must be a battalion of child psychiatric nurses, a company of education welfare officers, and the programme says there are some floats representing adolescent units, school 'refuges', special tutorial units, family therapy, behaviour therapy, occupational therapy and play therapy. Bringing up the rear are representatives of the staff of community homes, children's homes and hostels, special careers officers, officers of the juvenile courts, and finally members of various independent, philanthropic and voluntary organisations which help families and children.

This is admittedly a frivolous image and is not intended to imply that the resources for children in difficulties are generous. But it represents the immensely variegated and muddled arrangements that have developed over the years for boys and girls in difficulties. Attempts to define and co-ordinate services for children and adolescents even in a limited geographical area are characteristically bedevilled by confusion and uncertainty about who is doing what for whom. At an individual level the route a boy or girl takes to one expert or another is an extraordinarily arbitrary process.

Somehow child psychiatry perfuses this mixture. Theories of disorder and principles of treatment, developed by psychiatrists and psychologists of many persuasions, are used in many hundreds of different settings, sometimes in watered down, modified or misunderstood versions, sometimes applied with rigorous orthodoxy. Child psychiatrists themselves work in many different institutions and in quite different ways.

How can one make sense of this cacophony of experts and approaches? Undoubtedly specialists are needed, and a variety of services, but do we need so many? And how can they work together? It is not as if the variety is particularly to the advantage of children and their families. Variation there may be, but often to the extent that the adolescent unit or child guidance clinic serving district X takes a totally different approach to that serving district Y, and for the most part the population of each area is stuck with the service available. A social worker may be a first-rate family therapist, or run an excellent remedial drama group, but when he or she leaves for another office the service ceases. In many ways we seem to have the worst of both worlds, neither a true 'open market' of different sorts of skill provided by lots of individualistic professionals, nor a smoothly organised system in which every sort of service has its allotted place and the referral process to each is clear.

It is only too easy to be critical, and it is not the purpose of this book to beat people over the head and find fault, still less to join the fashionable anti-professional or anti-psychiatry bandwagons. Professionalism is important, but professionalism requires knowing what the job is, and where it ends, and many child psychiatrists *and* people who use, and encourage, child psychiatrists have not minded leaving the question of child psychiatry's limits rather open. Just because it is not easy to define the limits of psychiatry in any watertight way does not mean that the question should be dropped. Nor need any professional define his work with undue rigidity; but at least there should be some sort of consensus among child psychiatrists about the core of the specialty, and what its goals should be in day-to-day work and in the field's development. Again, because a consensus would be hard to reach does not mean that the matter should not be faced. Child psychiatry is an expensive commodity; the ingredients should be clearly marked on the label.

But child psychiatrists have not been willing to take more or less anything on particularly because of philanthropy or self-aggrandisement. The reasons are more complex.

Child psychiatry has provided two services to the community, one useful and one unhelpful if not disastrous. Helpfully, it has been a focus and a source of innovation for theory and for practice not only for different sorts of child psychiatrists, but for others interested in helping children. It has provided a meeting point for many different sorts of worker trying to understand in quite different ways how children grow and behave the way they do, and what can be done to enhance health and development and put right problems. For a long time the umbrella term 'psychiatry' has been regarded as a satisfactory general label for a wide range of work in which psychiatry (the medical study and treatment of mental disorder) has been in the minority. But the professions associated with child psychiatry, learning from it and contributing to it, have themselves developed and many are engaged in organising their own professional groups, training, examinations and so on. For their sake as well as child psychiatry's, the field of which child psychiatry has been the focus for so long needs critical reappraisal.

Unhelpfully, child psychiatry has also fulfilled a more atavistic function. Child psychiatrists are doctors, and doctors have traditionally been imbued with the authority to take on the impossible and have the last word (which also sanctions making mistakes), and allowed to be almost the last custodians of magic: who knows what medicine may not dream up, given the time and money? Brain transplants? Children and their families in the modern world present many painful dilemmas, ranging from the difficult to the impossible, and the peculiar medical mixture that endows child psychiatry, half magic and half scientific (just enough of each to maintain optimism), vaguely threatening and vaguely benevolent, has encouraged a large clientele of children with miscellaneous problems out of all proportion to its relative lack of success. Who can be satisfied with what we do about delinquency, mental retardation, or children without their own families? But if there is a psychiatrist to take a kindly interest in the most despondent of arrangements and establishments, like a priest visiting the poor, there is a feeling around that something is being done.

Child psychiatry being 'there' and sometimes doing nothing in particular has not only blurred the issue for child psychiatry, it has allowed areas in which child psychiatry has dabbled to become blurred too. There is, for example, nothing that child psychiatry can offer for the great majority of juvenile delinquents, but the hope that it might has led to all sorts of false starts in 'treatment'. It was right for child psychiatry to try, and equally right that it should withdraw; but where has it left those dealing with the problem? The ghost of the psychiatric presence is still around, with other professionals still wondering if someone else can 'cure' what child psychiatry couldn't.

A problem of a quite different sort affects all the professions dealing with children. Disturbed children make adults feel worried and guilty and anxious to be grown up and competent. We achieve equilibrium in different ways, depending on our backgrounds and personalities. There are the bluff and hearty, the earnest and obsessive, the relaxed, the fanatical, the modest and the charismatic, the scientific and the intuitive, the autocratic and the democratic, and somehow they have to work together. I do not think it is an exaggeration to say that inter-personal, inter-departmental and interprofessional ill-feeling, competition and rivalry is sufficiently evident to constitute quite a serious problem in child care. This is not because the people concerned are particularly wicked or neurotic. It is simply that the work is demanding, uncertainties considerable, disappointments frequent, and in general insufficient attention is given to dealing with the feelings generated between professionals in this work. People are drawn to the broad child care and treatment field for many different reasons, and many who are quite competent, or even excellent, in one aspect or another fall down in human relationships. There is no blueprint for coping with this inevitable clash of personalities, and those skilled in one or other of the psychotherapies are not noticeably exempt from experiencing or causing difficulty. But, as with the other problems mentioned, the matter deserves attention. No field is so full of emotional and inter-personal pitfalls, and none so full of people convinced that they personally really manage these matters rather well.

For these and other reasons there is room for improvement in the child care field, and what follows are personal views about what needs to be thought about and discussed as well as what needs to be done. To this extent a good deal of the argument is about services, and the ideal organisation of our work; if the discussion provokes thought about the curious way we organise and equip ourselves in order to help children in difficulties, it should also help generate ideas about how best to help individual boys and girls, and how to work with fellow professionals more productively. The central idea is contained in the title: how to use child psychiatry; and of course that means how to work with child psychiatrists. As the book is written from the viewpoint of a child and adolescent psychiatrist, the concepts of diagnosis and treatment used by many child and adolescent psychiatrists are emphasised. This is not in order to commend the psychiatric approach to members of other professions, but to explain what to expect, the possibilities and the limitations, if a boy or girl is referred to a psychiatric clinic. But by then, so to speak, it is too late, and the child has become a patient. The questions in the background, and which should recur in the following pages, are more fundamental: what's wrong? what's needed? who needs psychiatry? and who needs something else?

Conclusions

The broad child care and treatment field is growing in an extraordinarily rambling and incoherent way, and the service is patchy, with professions and facilities idiosyncratic in one area, duplicated in another and absent elsewhere. To some extent this is due to the very complicated and difficult social, psychological and biological problems with which people in the field are trying to contend. What is needed is not the imposition of bureaucratic attempts at 'organisation', which would, on past performance, finally gum up the works, but careful examination of the philosophy and function of each profession involved in relation to other professions, and in relation to children's needs.

2

Treatment, Training, Care or Control?

Late on a Friday afternoon, when everyone else has gone home, a social worker receives a telephone call from the children's home for which she is responsible. An anxious assistant residential care worker, new to the job and in charge for the weekend, is very worried about a girl of thirteen who has just hit one of the domestic staff and thrown her tea all over the floor. It emerges that the girl, who has been simmering all week, is now in a miserable rage. She became angry and upset following a visit from her father, whom she rarely sees, and demanded to go out. The last time something similar happened the girl bought some aspirins at a chemist's and took an overdose, and the residential worker does not want a recurrence. The other children, who caused a riot a month ago, and had begun to settle, are boiling up again because of the renewed tension in the home.

The domestic staff have had enough. If the girl isn't removed at once they will leave. The residential worker in charge feels much the same way after a tough week but can't say so. Her immediate colleagues are waiting for her to do something.

The child guidance clinic the girl once attended has been contacted but she cannot be seen there for at least a week. The children's home has a visiting child psychiatrist who isn't available. The social worker, having just spent most of two days trying to 'place' another girl

with an almost identical problem, knows that there is no
chance of finding somewhere else for her to go, even if
that was a good idea. Theoretically, if she had the time
and energy – which she hasn't – she could go into the
children's home and hold an emergency meeting of all
concerned to try to relieve feelings and sort things out.
However, both energy and time in abundance would be
needed because this is not the way that the home usually
operates. Moreover, the domestic staff in question have
already gone off and made it clear that they want the girl
out by the time they return. To complicate matters, the
residential worker does not particularly see eye-to-eye
with the warden of the children's home, an excellent but
independent-minded, middle-aged man, who in turn
doesn't get on too well with the social worker.

The girl *has* taken an overdose in the past, and is now
inaccessible to all reasonable approaches, and this, plus
the fact that her mother is reputedly in and out of
psychiatric hospitals, encourages the social worker to
suggest to the residential worker that the home's GP is
approached for help. Unfortunately, only a locum is on
duty in the practice, and knows no one at the children's
home. He is reluctant to get involved. Later, the
residential worker telephones the social worker to say
that the girl has wrecked her room and locked herself in
the bathroom, from which come the sounds of scream-
ing, running water and breaking glass. The GP now
comes, accompanied by an ambulance and two police
cars.

The girl, heavily sedated and now on a Section 29 of
the Mental Health Act, is whisked off to the local
general hospital casualty department, despite the angry
protests of the casualty department's Sister when she
heard what was on the way. The social worker now
telephones the local adolescent psychiatric unit. All the
staff there are in a meeting because of a crisis to do with
one of their girls: but they're full up in any case, says the
secretary. The area adult psychiatric hospital is con-

tacted; the registrar on duty says, yes, send her in, but
he will have to confirm it first with the duty consultant,
and comes back with a very firm 'No'; the girl is too
young; the hospital has had a lot of adverse criticism for
admitting an adolescent a year ago; they don't admit
anybody under seventeen; in any case, the admission
ward is very disturbed and full of elderly people.

Meanwhile the girl is wide awake and abusing the
nursing staff who have had to tie her hands; the physician
in charge of the casualty department has been contacted
by the Sister, and is now on the telephone to the social
worker demanding that something be done at once.

The psychiatric unit of the general hospital itself? This
suggestion earns a massive broadside: too young, too
disturbed, full up, on a Section too near the children's
surgical ward, can't get hold of a psychiatrist at the
weekend, only the radiotherapy house physician on duty,
he's new, he's a locum, etc.

Back to the adolescent unit; no chance at all of an
emergency admission, even if it was appropriate. Offer of
an assessment next week.

Most social workers are familiar with this sort of situation; those who aren't have it to look forward to. It is also
well known that this sort of crisis doesn't go away or blow
over. The child's fury and despair goes on and on, as very
often it has done for years, although not always expressed
as openly as in this sort of outburst. The thinly-stretched
staff in the children's home, with no way of easing the
pain of the situation, are in a similar difficult position to
those in the three psychiatric units contacted, and in the
other children's homes that could not take her in; no one
knows what answer to give the girl who is raging that no
one knows how to look after her, because she is right.
The only magical hope in the back of the minds of many
involved is the breathing space earned by a syringeful of
sedative – for the girl, of course.

This example illustrates a number of themes taken up in more detail later.

1   During this crisis who is responsible for this young girl? Who should be looking after her?
2   Is she mentally ill?
3   Various professionals and organisations are being approached; what can they do that the children's home staff can't?
4   What are the adults in this vignette up to? The stereotype of the worker in this field is that of the cool, competent, kind professional. No one seems to fit this portrait here.
5   How have things got this way for this girl? What is she doing in a children's home? What are the staff trying to do? What is there about all the people involved – girl, children's home staff, social worker, psychiatrist and others – that can allow this girl to become, one Friday evening, a 'hot potato' nobody wants to handle? What on earth does she make of it? or has she learned to take such adult behaviour for granted?

Responsibility for the girl

To appreciate the extent to which the young person here is being let down by adults, it is worth comparing the situation with a less emotive example.

A small boy develops vomiting and abdominal pain, and his parents call the family doctor who diagnoses acute appendicitis and sends the boy to hospital. After a brief examination, an operation and a short period of convalescence, the boy returns home. Throughout, responsibility is clear. His parents remain responsible for him, and part of exercising this responsibility includes entrusting aspects of his care, for a time, to professionals (family doctor, surgeon, nurses) who can do something they cannot. The child understands this. He will be frightened and perhaps tearful at times and no doubt, given the choice, would not want to go to hospital or have treatment. Nevertheless his parents, trusting the medical and surgical opinions, have no qualms about exercising their parental authority and sharing in a kindly and firm insistence that treatment is carried out. Nor is there undue delay in arranging it. Even if things do not go totally smoothly, e.g. the doctor is an unfamiliar locum, the hospital scruffy, the surgical registrar brusque and the ward Sister grudging about parental visiting, there is nevertheless a feeling, justified by events, that a necessary technical job has been done well enough, and after a week or two the child and family can continue their lives. The only scars are abdominal ones.

The situation with the girl in the children's home is quite different. The 'medical model' has been clumsily attempted, in that a case has been made that the girl is 'ill' and should be removed to a place of treatment, but this is not adhered to with conviction. Thus, had the children's home staff agreed to cope for a few more days, or the local reception centre found a place for her, the social worker would probably have been as grateful for this as for a hospital place. The latter might have been the local adult hospital, or an adolescent unit, but the social worker's main concern could well have been to get the girl from A to B rather than to be concerned with the details of what happens when she gets there. This is not to say that the social worker would not be concerned if the child was accepted by an institution with a grim reputation, and indeed he or she might block that move. But even in an adolescent unit psychiatric care is much more of an unknown quantity with uncertain results than is, say, surgery for appendicitis. Why, then, does the social worker, whose integrity there is no reason to doubt, seem willing to take this step?

There are four hypothetical answers. One is that the girl's behaviour is genuinely regarded as a problem more likely to be helped by psychiatric treatment than by anything else. Second, there is the belief that when someone is behaving inexplicably, uncontrollably, or both, psychiatrists have effective ways of stopping them. Third, when children and adolescents suddenly become beyond control, there are three well trodden paths: to a children's reception centre; the police station and thence to a remand centre; or to hospital. Finally, an anxiety and despair-laden feeling that when things are awful hospitals should help.

' What these facilities have to offer is not however clear. What the police might have done is increasingly blurred by an overlap with social work; what the social services department might have achieved in their reception centre, namely looking after the child, is muddled with concepts of 'therapy'; and, most obscure of all, what the psychiatric unit might do is conveniently blurred so that whether the child ultimately returns to the children's home, goes on to another, or stays in the psychiatric unit for years, becomes an open question and one left to a considerable extent to the hospital team. This is not because the child care staff don't care about the young person concerned, but because a) their own resources for dealing with troubled children are so thinly stretched that anything, even hospital, is preferable, and b) because the reasons for admission aren't clear, and, as mentioned earlier, 'proper looking after' and 'therapy' have somehow been allowed to become blurred and even synonymous. It is as if the proper but temporary and qualified sharing of parental responsibility with technically expert outsiders (as in the case of the child with appendicitis) has become a grossly distorted parody of medical help. As a result the seeking of psychiatric help and advice (which is reasonable enough) has been transformed by panic and uncertainty into a situation where the child's home and education and current relationships are placed in jeopardy. She's 'had to go to hospital'.

Is the girl mentally ill?

Mental illness is difficult to define with precision. The
problem is often that, when in doubt, if a child is hard to
manage and emotionally troubled, the assumption is
made that the 'emotional disorder' must be treated first,
then he or she can be looked after properly. Very often
the reverse is the case; with proper looking after,
'disorder' disappears. Of course, with mental illness
being so hard to pin down as an entity, it would be
perfectly right for psychiatric team and care workers to
get together and in a systematic way talk through the
girl's troubles with her and between themselves, and
plan the necessary work together. And indeed this often
happens; but not in an emergency like this one, where
the assumption has already been made that there is
something wrong in the girl's head.

Psychoanalysts and biochemists and others do of
course have theoretical models whereby things can go
wrong in the head. For many sociologists the supposed
mechanisms of behavioural functioning and the mind
are mystifying red herrings drawing people's attention
away from the economic and social forces which really
shape their thinking, conveniently, it is alleged, for
mental health professionals. Between these extremes
are many conceptual models of mental functioning and
abnormality – some biological, some to do with the way
small groups and families operate together, some based
on the principles of behavioural psychology.

The term, 'mental illness' means thought, feeling and
behaviour which is abnormal a) being inappropriate for
the circumstances and b) causing distress, disability or
both. It is clear that this is no watertight definition; who
decides what is or isn't appropriate, for example? If we
had a clear conception of normal mental functioning
then mental illness could be defined along such lines.
Certainly there are extremes of mental abnormality such
as grossly disordered thinking patterns, clouded con-

sciousness, grossly abnormal beliefs adhered to with conviction ('I *know*, without doubt, that my recent run of bad luck was plotted by men from space who have moved into the flat upstairs'), extreme depression with social withdrawal, and gross euphoria and excitement that justify the term illness, but these are not common.

Mental illness, and the 'milder' term, emotional disorder, both carry the connotation of individual disorder. It is important to distinguish this if one can from a child's manifest anxiety, despair or lack of confidence being quite clearly caused and sustained by the way the adults in his life are handling him. It is unreasonable to 'diagnose' a child as emotionally disordered if the change needed is not in the child but in the way he or she is being handled. (One may perhaps describe a child, conveniently ambiguously, as 'disturbed', without prejudging who is doing the disturbing.)

The girl in the example might have turned out to be acutely ill, e.g. with a manic depressive or schizophrenic illness. This would be exceedingly rare. Much more common would be the situation where a girl who has never felt properly looked after over the years therefore becomes increasingly unhappy and angry, and finds that the adults trying to look after her find her a nuisance, a problem, and a worry rather than a rewarding child. She continues to have childish rages, and opportunities for ordinary social learning and reciprocation of affection get pushed to one side. A vicious circle develops in which the child is less and less rewarding, more and more impulsive and despairing, and with child and adults forced together because of circumstances rather than drawn together by mutual interest and affection. The only way out of this impasse is for adults to find the child's behaviour worth putting up with for her own sake. This is a lot to ask, and she senses this. If this is an adequate description of this girl's problem, there seems no reason to invoke the concept of mental illness. Descriptively she shows emotional disturbance, but a child in this predicament would be expected to. She needs proper looking after, and this needs to be distinguished from psychotherapy, even if the exercise is a difficult one.

At what point does this girl's unhappy way of reacting become part of her own make-up, and less dependent on the immediate circumstances? It is hard to say, but certainly at that point she can be said to 'have' a disorder. Whether it is 'psychiatric' is another matter.

What can the experts do that the children's home can't?

The process of referral embodies two quite different types of expectation. First, the wish to be helped in a general way, e.g. by reassurance, encouragement or (as in this case) by being relieved of responsibility for what looks like an impossible situation. Second, the assumption that the specialists to whom referral is made have the experience and resources to carry out a necessary technical job, as embodied in the case of the child with appendicitis.

Perhaps the most useful aspect of the referral, as far as the staff involved are concerned, would be the opportunity to encapsulate, and thereby bring some control to, a chaotic situation by getting an outsider to take an overall view of what is going on. The very act of seeking another's help means that those doing so have acknowledged being in difficulties and needing something from 'outside', and this alone is a crisis of sorts, and an important therapeutic step for whoever is in trouble, including the girl. The ability to seek help is a skill enhanced by experience and maturity. In this example, the *girl's* way of seeking help is immature, chaotic and likely to drive it away.

As for technical expertise, there is certainly a core of accumulating knowledge and technique in child and adolescent psychiatry which justifies its position as a

specialist resource. Many child psychiatrists, by training, inclination and because they tend to work with
colleagues in related professions, are able to take a broad
view of the problems presented to them. They ought,
therefore, to be able to make an accurate assessment of
the child and situation. Similarly, a child psychiatrist
and his or her team are in a strong position to recommend what course of action is likely to help. Here,
however, is where a distinction appears which may turn
out to be a helpful division of labour or a problematic
split: psychiatric assessment may help but *treatment* as
such has its limitations, and this varies of course from
child to child. For a very small minority, it is right for a
child psychiatric team to take over more or less completely. For the majority, however, a great deal remains
to be done for the child which people outside the
psychiatric team can do best.

What a child psychiatric team can actually do is the
subject of a later chapter. Meanwhile, the answer to the
question 'what can the experts do that the children's
home can't?' is: sometimes a great deal, but almost
always there is a lot that can and should be done by those
who already have the responsibility for looking after the
young person concerned.

But surely, some may argue, there would be nothing
wrong with a wildly disturbed child whom no one can
control going off in an emergency to hospital, being put
to bed, sedated if necessary, and returned as soon as she
cools down to the children's home? Certainly there can
be a place for this sort of response, for example when a
child like the girl described above needs to be given a
message along these lines by the child care staff:

We care about you and what happens to you and are
going to provide all we can for you for the next few
years; but sometimes you push us too far, hitting
people and smashing things up, and we then can't
cope by ourselves. When you get like that all we can

do is put you somewhere that can manage that sort of behaviour one way or another until you cool down and it's time to come home again and carry on where we left off.

This can be an excellent arrangement for some young people where a long-term home (including of course their natural home) is able and willing to work with the child through his or her long-term problems in emotional development. It can operate when, say, a good children's home and a unit staffed for such crises (not necessarily a hospital, incidentally) are used to working together, or carefully plan a special arrangement of this sort in a particular child's case. But the essence of the arrangement is to *enable the people at the children's home to carry on working with the child*, and in practice it is quite difficult to hold and reverse the process by which, for years, the child has learned that each new home is without hope and the best thing to do is to try another. The risks, often materialising, are that the girl 'settles down' in hospital and the home fades into the background, or that both home and hospital give up and the girl goes on to other homes and hospitals. To repeat the point made earlier: some such plan, carefully thought out, could be just what is needed; but such plans tend not to be made, and quasi-'psychiatric' emergencies allowed to blow up instead.

What is happening among the adults?

Under pressure, people tend to regress, which is a technical way of saying that because of anxiety or despair they return to a more immature way of coping. This does not necessarily take the form of 'going to pieces'. The cool detachment of a doctor writing a prescription before the patient has finished speaking can be an immature defence; conversely getting heated and angry can sometimes be the right professional response. Children, especially disturbed children, generate conflicting feelings in adults trying to look after them; the powerful desire to help can compete with an equally powerful wish to get them off one's back. It is difficult to get on with the job in the face of such competing feelings and different people make individual adjustments to them, so that the compromise some staff reach is to be that much more sympathetic while others adjust in the direction of being less so.

Among adults looking after a disturbed and challenging child the following will often be happening:

(a) They are not listening to each other
The various people involved or half-involved are acting on catch phrases like 'acutely disturbed', 'cannot cope', without knowing the anxieties of the people asking for help nor the resources of the people whose help is sought.

(b) Anxiety
Nothing undermines capacity to cope with a problem more effectively than the suspicion, or knowledge, that there is no need to press on. Anxiety is inevitable in coping with the girl's behaviour but other nagging doubts are now being added; are we (in the children's home), the right people for the job? Will we be held responsible if serious damage is done? Will our colleagues and seniors support us if things go wrong? If there are no domestic staff to clean up and cook breakfast in the morning, what will we do? Who will get the blame? Furthermore, when such crises have temporarily blown over, is it at the expense of one or two staff who are left feeling terrible, and apprehensive about the next time? With half the staff pressing for the girl's removal, quite possibly supported by the children's home warden, and the social worker feeling the responsibility for maintaining what he or she thinks are good relationships with the staff, all the pressures are on for the girl's removal, and few for her to stay.

(c) **Competition**

The adults involved are not motivated only by avoidance of anxiety. There is also disagreement about who knows best. When children and adolescents challenge adults to look after them there is an inevitable difference in parenting and care-taking style from adult to adult. If the disagreement is discussed openly, the very fact of acknowledging the gaps helps bridge them. If denied, the anxious child will force the adults farther apart and put them into competition and conflict with each other as surely as night follows day. People then start blaming each other and do not draw together again unless *either* they idealise some outside agency which will solve these apparently insoluble problems, *or* someone within the organisation or outside is blamed for all the pain. Getting together for either reason will not help the girl, though the adults may feel better.

(d) **Despair and uncertainty about what to do**

Skill, knowledge and experience are needed as well as good intentions. This means not only skill in understanding the girl's feelings and her relationships with adults, but also understanding the relationships between staff.

There are problems here. Even elementary knowledge about how best to look after children is unevenly distributed. There are wise old people who, with a wink, show they know what to do and indeed run excellent establishments until they retire. There are also people new to the job who have read or heard something psychoanalytic or sociological about the game which may not match the problems they are faced with, but who resort readily to jargon and techniques which irritate their colleagues. The supervisory and training machinery for looking at what they are doing, day to day, and learning from it, may be absent or scanty. Although there are sound principles which can be acquired from books and didactic teaching, skilful management of disturbed children depends also on skills in working with other people, rather than on implementing set management schemes and trendy techniques. As well as training and intelligence it requires dealing with feelings, other people's as well as one's own, and this includes skill in giving and using support. All this requires time. In the example, the children's home has not invested enough time or resources into questions of the girl's needs, what she has provoked in the staff, and how they should respond. Perhaps there are too few staff, for example, to contemplate setting time aside for discussing what sort of a job they are doing. Many institutions regard this as a luxury they can't afford, which is one of the most myopic and false economies imaginable, and a common one too.

How have things developed this way for this girl?

The proposals being made on her behalf are that she is mentally ill and would be better off in hospital. Analysis of her predicament at any level – commonsensical or sophisticated – suggests that the most likely explanation is that for many years the girl has, with justification, not felt properly looked after, and so much time and energy has been spent in provoking and challenging grown ups to look after her that a) she has remained impatient, untrusting, impulsive and angry and b) the nicer things that go on between children and adults have never become established in her personal repertoire or domestic setting. This explanation points to a solution: proper looking after, education and training. But her feelings and behaviour make it increasingly difficult for this to be set up and sustained. What has happened is attempt after attempt by more and more 'specialised' people to hold her in the sense that a small

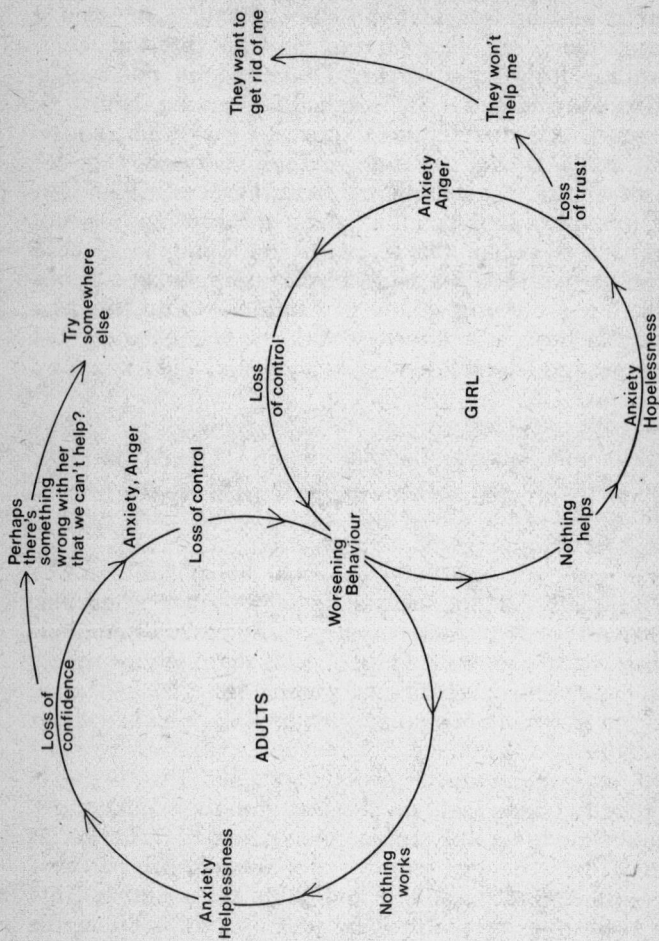

Fig. 1 Deteriorating relationships and the beginning of a further move.

child needs to be held. Her parents couldn't provide affection and social training and so were joined by the social worker, but nor could they do this together. The social worker therefore placed her in a children's home but this broke down too, so she moved to another, changing schools in the process, and then ceased to be manageable in either school or the new home. She was put in a boarding school for maladjusted pupils but left after a series of crises and was found another where things went wrong too. Expelled with little notice, she was placed in a children's home on an emergency basis and then moved to another, and then another. Sometimes her moves have been to a school or home where there was supposedly more skill, sometimes, particularly in emergencies, to the only place available. Unfortunately all this is far from uncommon in our handling of children.[104, 105, 114, 115]

Chapter 3 outlines the foundations required for proper development. In terms of emotional development the childhood of the girl in this example has hardly begun, though chronologically it is nearly over.

It may be felt that this example, with the extreme reactions of both the girl and the professional workers, bears little resemblance to day-to-day matters in child care and child psychiatry. In fact there are fields of work, particularly with adolescents, where this sort of situation is far from uncommon. More important, however, is the fact that many lesser problems can be handled less efficiently and less kindly because of very similar misunderstandings and personal and inter-personal difficulties. The child who is referred to a psychiatrist because no one else has time to talk to him, or because the child is making a nuisance of himself and the path to the psychiatric clinic is a well-trodden one; the problem which is perceived as a psychiatric problem because of lack of knowledge of child development, or of what child psychiatrists do; the child moved from a school or children's home because of anxieties and embarrassment about mildly deviant behaviour and the lack of anyone on the staff who can cope with it, or because disagreement about the child is setting members of staff against each other; the child who does indeed need psychiatric help, and gets it, but whose parents and teachers withdraw somewhat, or more than somewhat, from their responsibilities to the child until he or she is 'cured'.

Conclusion: treatment, training, care or control?

All children need *care*. This means a sense of security of tenure with a group of other people – usually the family – which includes adults competent enough and sufficiently interested to provide food, warmth, affection, stimulation, and the dawning experience that sharing life with them is a worthwhile exercise despite inevitable conflicts, anxieties and disappointments.

All children need *training and education*, including upbringing according to the rules of reasonable social behaviour and the development of academic, social and creative skills to the child's potential. The ability to *play*[112] is a literally vital capacity which grows out of proper care and education.

If care or education has been inadequate, special care and special education are needed, how much depending on the degree of deficiency. As to the question of who should provide it, with experience, help and advice, parents and 'ordinary' teachers can concentrate on special areas of difficulty in a child's growth, learning and creativity, and this may be sufficient. Sometimes the help of specially trained professionals is needed, for example social workers and remedial teachers.

All children need *control*. Setting limits on behaviour is complementary to care and education. Getting the balance right between allowing the child to experiment, and persuading him or her to do not this but that, is a fundamental skill of competent parents and teachers. Again, if a child is unfortunate enough for his parents' and teachers' skills to be inadequate, more specialised professionals are drawn in. Leaving out the middle ground (social workers, teachers in schools for the 'maladjusted') the boy or girl who is allowed to get away with an ever wider range of misbehaviour ends up with the police, the courts, the probation services and ultimately may get locked up.[47,66]

The word *treatment*, or its more elegant euphemism *therapy*, is quite often applied to special methods of care, education and control, which is a pity because this usage is potentially misleading. This field is full enough of complications, obscurities and misunderstandings without adding to them. I would like to persuade the reader that, for the sake of clarity, the word treatment should be confined to a small but important area, the correction of disorder. The fact that it is not easy to draw a line between, say, problems in developing a linguistic skill and a disorder of language, or naughtiness and 'conduct disorder' does not mean that we should give up the attempt to clarify the emphasis of what we are trying to do for a particular boy or girl: treatment, training/ education care or control.

This is as important in the planning and development of services for boys and girls in trouble as it is in the case of the individual child. All children need care, education and control, and some need special care, education and control. Not many children, fortunately, need treatment but when they do provision must be made for their care, education and control too. 'Therapists' shouldn't do it all: others do it better.

In the example with which this chapter began, the girl's first need is for care and control. Without control, neither she, nor the adults looking after her, will feel safe. Control in this context does not necessarily mean

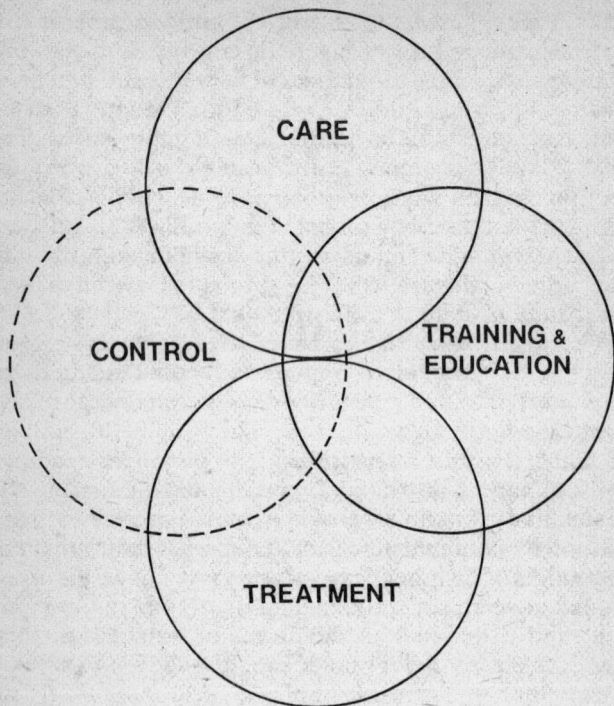

Fig. 2 Treatment, training (and education), care and control. *NB Treatment* incorporates elements of control and training but it does not replace them. *Treatment* and *care* are quite distinct.

physical security; it can also mean sufficient mature adults able to trust themselves and each other to limit firmly the girl's behaviour without giving up, and this is not an easy task. It requires training, supervision and support, which in turn require time and space and these are expensive, although probably not as expensive as hospitals would have to be to do the same job, *if* this was a good idea. The fact that care and control are breaking down in the example given does not by itself mean that she needs treatment instead.

Conclusions

In this chapter, specialist expertise has been defined in terms of successively more specialised degrees of professionalism. Thus, if a teacher cannot meet a child's educational needs, the boy or girl is passed on to a more specialised teacher with the time and experience to focus on the learning disability. Similarly with successive attempts at control, ending with prison. Psychiatry, and therefore child psychiatry, is in a quite different position, or should be. In practice people turn to psychiatry for dealing with extremes of behaviour, characteristically as a last resort. Psychiatry has got itself into this role for historical reasons, with consequences that do more harm than good. When care, education and control fail, what is needed is better care, education and control. Psychiatric treatment should be reserved for psychiatric disorder, and should be an option, not a last resort.

3

The Development of Children and the Emergence of Problems

How child development is conceptualised

An account of the theories of child development would be a lengthy distraction, but an outline of the concepts used in understanding normal and abnormal development will put the following chapters into perspective. A good deal of confusion is caused because child psychiatrists give the impression that it is right to adhere to a particular school of thought. Most would deny that they do, and claim to be eclectic. The fact is that in practice many psychiatrists do decide rather early in their professional life (and indeed early in the life of a speciality which is hardly sixty years old) that one particular way of looking at human development is the right one. Other professions are just as bad.

Human development isn't simple. A child develops physically, emotionally, intellectually and socially and moreover the child affects the feelings and behaviour and therefore the responses of those around him.[87] These responses, in turn, affect the further development of the child. But the ways in which adults respond are also influenced by their own experiences, past and current. Parents' and teachers' responses to the child therefore depend partly on their own personalities, but also on the cultural setting in which they operate.

Understanding a child's state – normal or abnormal –

at any given time (e.g. at the point of referral) requires appreciation that the matters to be considered are:

> *Multiple*
> *Developing and changing*
> *Interacting with each other, not isolated*
> *Dynamic, not static*

Multiple factors

Consider an unhappy boy of seven brought with dragging feet by his mother to the doctor's surgery. He is a bed wetter. Is there 'something wrong' with him? One could jump to conclusions and assume that we have here evidence of a child with a disturbed mind, showing his problem by wetting the bed. Another practitioner might be inclined to feel that his mother is over-anxious, or that the child has an abnormal bladder. A family therapist might wonder what family problem was being expressed by the wet sheets.

Fig. 3 shows the multiple ways in which all people operate all the time. There is adequate material for every school of thought; how can it be decided which sort of explanation is correct? It helps to be aware at least of the range of possibilities.

Bed wetting, and its recognition as a 'problem' varies widely from culture to culture (C) and indeed from community to community within one country (S).[94] Moving down the level of the diagram, the doctor's reputation in the neighbourhood will influence the mother's decision whether or not to take the boy along once she has decided that his behaviour is not right. But so might washing and drying facilities in that particular area: the nuisance value of recurrent wet sheets and bed wetting as a problem, is likely to vary with the availability of washing machines, gardens etc. for dealing with them (N). What the person using the next machine in the Launderama has to say about the implications of

Fig. 3   Levels of functioning.

C *Cultural:*	Beliefs and expectations in a country or ethnic group about what is normal and abnormal, and how deviations are labelled and dealt with. E.g. notions of good and bad, right and wrong, healthy and unhealthy.
S *Social:*	As above but in a narrower context: social class, age group, material resources, availability of services and access to them.
N *Neighbourhood:*	Immediate attitudes, pressures and expectations among friends, neighbours, teachers, acquaintances; local environmental conditions: schools, parks, roads, gardens.
F *Family:*	Family attitudes and beliefs, parental strengths and weaknesses, ability to nurture and show affection, stimulate, encourage, respond to distress, set limits, teach and to enable appropriate degrees of autonomy among its members.
B *Behaviour:*	What the child actually does: act aggressively, look depressed or frightened, wet the bed, eat or not eat, talk or not talk, play, speech, social skills.
P *Psyche:*	How the child thinks and learns, what he or she believes and feels, and what we infer the child feels but can't directly express. Intellectual level, developmental skills and emotional life.
T *Temperamental, constitutional and physical:*	Qualities partly inherited and partly determined by early experiences; physical disease or disabilities; sex differences; the more physiological aspects of development and intellectual functioning.

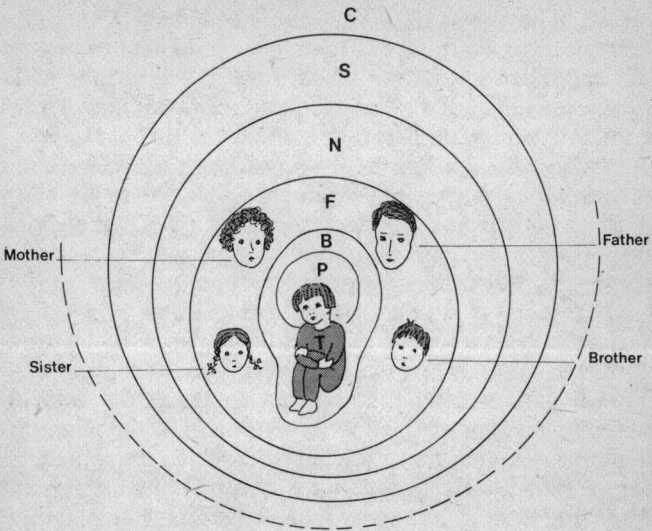

bed wetting in a seven year old boy may also be a factor in the referral.

Next, whatever may be the origins in the family of this boy's enuresis, his bed wetting will affect the family somehow. Will it be a shameful secret kept from father? Or from the other siblings? Will it be kept from the neighbours? It may well be a cause of more anxiety in one family than another. It often runs in families; the parents' memories of his or her own childhood enuresis will affect the parental response, with an effect on the child that may provoke or allay anxiety. And what might mother-in-law say? She may have firm views about her daughter-in-law's ability to bring up children.

Then there is the child's own behaviour (B) and psyche or mental life (P). When does he wet the bed and why? The boy may have an emotional problem (a minority of enuretics, about a quarter, do); or he may be growing up normally but under a current additional stress. The immediate situation may affect the child's behaviour too, thus enuresis characteristically ceases during short spells away from home, beginning again on the child's return. And anxiety about enuresis may in turn interfere with learning bladder control.

Finally, the child's neuro-physiological and general physical health and development (T) need to be considered. Disorders of the bladder (of which the most important is perhaps urinary infection in girls) may be the cause, but this is unusual.[94]

Distinct from disease of the bladder is the concept of variation in development. All children begin by wetting at night, and over the next few years the incidence falls. This boy is wetting his bed, but so are 20 per cent of other seven year olds. In what sense is this abnormal? It depends on what the clinician finds when he considers the various 'levels' of functioning shown in the diagram. The only abnormality may be a statistical one.

Development and change

One aspect therefore of assessing the situation is to look at how things *are*. Another, which requires a different sort of thinking, is to see how they are developing. The ability to conceptualise change, including differential change, over time is essential in understanding any living system. A gardener will not be interested only in how a young sapling looks one bleak Tuesday afternoon in November; he will picture how it has grown since he planted it, and the possible effect of varying weather and soil conditions, past and future, and how it might look in relation to other aspects of the garden, also constantly changing with the seasons and the years. This does not mean that immediate plant physiology is unimportant, but that the skilled gardener has to think in terms of past and future developments as well as how things are this week. And children's lives are more complicated than those of cabbages.

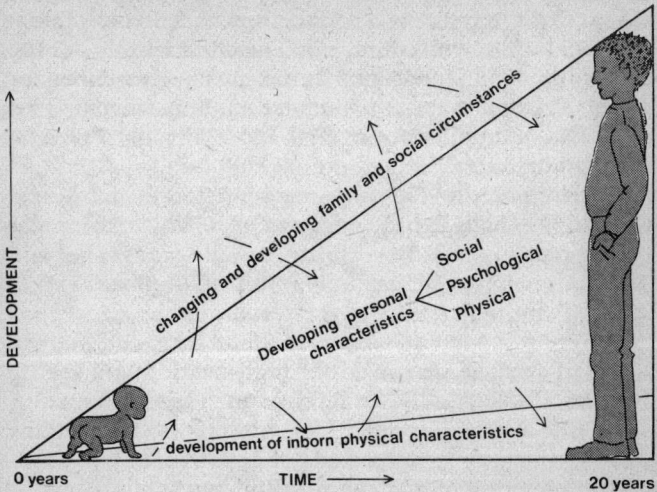

Fig. 4 Change and interaction over time. The arrows represent the way in which personal social, psychological and physical characteristics develop out of the interaction between innate characteristics and external social and other circumstances.

All seven levels described above are changing but they don't change at the same pace, and there is variation from individual to individual. Ideas of socially accepted behaviour change just as the body grows and changes over the years. Families develop new strengths and also run into periods of difficulties. They accumulate new members and lose old ones.

As the child *develops physically* he or she acquires the familiar 'milestones' of growth: bladder and bowel control, talking and walking, playing and the beginning of social skills and the ability to converse. These capacities are partly inborn but are also modified by what each child experiences. Some experiences enhance latent potential, others discourage it. The child with his or her individual predispositions is progressively shaped by many deliberate and accidental circumstances. This applies as much to personality and skills as to physiological attributes.

Intellectual development – capacity for thinking and reasoning – and the *acquisition of skills*, like motor co-ordination and the ability to use language and calculation, proceed similarly, with neurophysiological capacity influenced to a greater or lesser degree by experience of the outside world. Perceiving and making sense of what is perceived through hearing and seeing develop differentially, different functions maturing at different stages. Piaget[71,72,73] described the child's successive capacity, as periods of growth are reached, to reason in different and more skilful ways.

Emotional development is almost impossible to outline without reference to a number of quite different schools of thought. I have outlined a simplified scheme for emotional development in the following pages, borrowing from different authorities I have found helpful, particularly Klein,[53] Erikson,[29,30] Bowlby,[8,9,10,11] and Winnicott,[111,112,113] all of whom owe much to Freud.[34,96] What they have in common is the assumption that at each stage in development the individual can only make sense of, and react to, new experiences, demands, opportunities and stresses, in the light of his total experience so far. This may seem an unremarkable proposition. What has provoked disagreement is that psychoanalytical thinking maintains that feelings and fantasies of which the child is *largely unconscious* continue to influence conscious behaviour and reactions, even in adult life. For example, a girl copes with an impossibly unreliable and inconsistent father by idealising him and years later (unconsciously) chooses as a husband a superficially 'ideal' man who turns out to have her father's faults. But what a thing to admit! The psychoanalytic approach, not surprisingly, provokes love or hate.

Behavioural psychology has a quite different approach, although, in my view, one that is not inconsistent with psychoanalytic theory if the former says 'how' and the latter 'why'. It supposes the progressive shaping of the child's patterns of feeling, thinking and behaviour by the effect of external factors which selectively encourage, discourage, reward and punish the child's responses. The child smiles and makes noises, and mother beams and responds; the child learns, without being aware of it (although behaviour theorists tend to deny unconscious processes), that smiling and making noises are the things to do.

Social learning and child-parental interaction link these approaches. A useful critical review of various psychological and biological views of the interaction between developing children and their parents is Rutter's *Maternal Deprivation Reassessed*,[79] while Bowlby's writings on attachment theory[8, 9, 10, 11] provide conceptual models for individual growth through interaction and experiences with parents.

Interaction of developmental with other factors A boy may have inherited a sort of bladder that matures later rather than sooner. Suppose full bladder control would become established, normally for him, at around six or seven. Since the continent habit is newly established it is vulnerable for a time, and the child's anxiety when he notices his parents having a number of quite painful arguments results in loss of control again. His mother, ashamed of the rows (F), fearful of marital breakdown because of her own childhood experience (and because marital breakdown now seems so common (C.S.)) is too anxious to mention this to the doctor, who prescribes a bell and pad for the boy and, in due course, a tranquilliser for his mother. Had the marital discord occurred when the child was three or four, or when he became nine or ten and with well established bladder control, enuresis might never have happened. Divorce, maternal depression, school refusal, conduct disorder, learning difficulties at school or indeed nothing serious at all, might have been the result. But this pattern of events, in this sequence, at this time, resulted in enuresis.

Dynamic interaction   This is yet another dimension of development and interaction. The term 'dynamic' is borrowed from mechanical science and refers to movement and change (or the apparent lack of it) as a result of various forces operating in different directions. Perhaps the simplest example is the constancy of the water level in the bath if the plug is out and the tap sufficiently open. Many apparently static states in psychiatry may be the outcome of conflicting forces. For example a common source of dispute is that of adolescent 'rebelliousness'. Careful pieces of research have demonstrated that most adolescents are not particularly overtly rebellious against their parents.[84] On the other hand, scepticism, testing-out, anger, argument and verbal or physical aggression is frequent among 'disturbed' and delinquent adolescents, and indeed among groups of adolescents who have not actually broken the law, when adult controls are removed, as is seen in street disturbances when community authority breaks down. Is such behaviour qualitatively different from normal adolescent behaviour, or does it represent the release of a normal adolescent potential for rebelliousness when internal or external controls are removed or inadequate? The psychodynamic viewpoint would be the latter, and the conforming adolescents of the reported survey evidence either of the equilibrating effect of a good family and culture, or of 'repression'. Anthropological thinking, and Winnicott among others,[113] suggest that the adolescent passage to adulthood cannot conceivably be negotiated without questioning and challenging the adult world, and that this is not a cool and rational exercise but one accompanied by a great deal of heat. But of course we are talking about one aspect of a dynamic process, and this potential for rage and rebellion may normally be met and coped with by psychological and cultural forces. When the latter fail, the anger of the 'disturbed' boy or girl is understandable in terms of what was hitherto only one of a number of competing forces.

Observable and concrete factors also interact in a dynamic sense. Thus, over the years, a boy and his father may have furious rows with each other which only become threatening as the boy becomes more articulate than his father and then approaches and overtakes him in physique.

Families change too. The problems of a pubescent girl being flirtatious towards her father would be coped with safely in most families, but in a particular case, where for example the parents' marital or sexual relationship was in difficulties, anxiety about incest and marital breakdown might be so near the surface as to make it impossible for mother and father calmly, together and with appropriate humour, to get the girl to stop. Frequently discussion about adolescent 'crises', real or imagined, ignore the fact that at about that age the parents are often moving from relative youth to middle-age, and losing their own parents, and this too can upset the dynamic equilibrium a family has achieved.

Emotional development as an unfolding story

The roots of personality development are to be found well before conception, in the genetic predispositions to certain aspects of neurophysiological functioning and development that the child will inherit, and in the wishes, hopes and fears in the family about the sort of child the baby will turn out to be. These anticipations grow with the baby in the womb, and form the foundation of all sorts of fulfilled ambitions and frustrated hopes yet to come.

There is accumulating evidence about the influence on the child of the birth and what follows immediately. In the past there has been a great deal of misunderstanding about 'traumatic experiences' affecting a child in later life. There is no good evidence of the powerful impact of single emotional experiences, but it does seem that cumulative experiences can shape and direct a child in a particular direction,[86, 87] and indeed it would be surprising if this were not so.

A mouse running across a pregnant woman's abdomen will not produce mouse phobia in the child, though this has been one of many favourite old wives' tales. But consider the experience of an articulate and healthy middle-class woman and her husband, both fresh from ante-natal clinics and classes, the child within checked and double-checked and topped up with necessary nutrients, welcome friends and relatives skilfully kept standing by and unhelpful ones at a distance. The couple are hardly aware that they are using their considerable social skills to get the best out of the doctors, nurses and the whole confinement. Compare this with an inarticulate, hard-up girl of seventeen, angrily told by the tetchy midwife to put out that cigarette, this is a hospital you know, anxiously awaiting the arrival of her nervous and scruffy boyfriend on his motorbike from the pub, where with his mates he has been drowning his sorrows. She has missed many ante-natal clinics and most classes, wishes her mum would hurry up and arrive but the buses are unreliable. From what she thinks a doctor murmured to a nurse, there might be something wrong with the baby, but she didn't like to ask, they're so kind but they're all so busy. The first baby goes off home early in the company Cortina, the second baby is whisked away even earlier to the special care unit.

It is not as if such experiences directly affect the baby one way or another. But in the mother's contact with the baby, the support she has from her husband, the skill with which professional staff do enough but not too much, the child's fitness and responsiveness, the mother's mood, confidence and ability to take charge of her baby and feed, hold and stimulate the child with skill, the seeds are sown for the sort of toddler, and infant, and adolescent the boy or girl might be, and the dice loaded one way or another for the sort of family and neighbourhood and school he or she may grow up in. None of these are absolutes, but they are powerful, accumulative pressures gently easing a boy or girl in a particular direction as the early years go by.

From the first, what does the child make of it? Nothing, of course. There isn't a thought or a memory in his head. Of all the theories of child development, some aspects of the picture painted by Melanie Klein,[53, 118] are convincing because it is hard to imagine the world of the child possibly being anything else. Initially, a meaningless chaos of sensations coming and going, and not the slightest reason why the child's dawning consciousness should distinguish, or be able to distinguish, what is his and what comes from outside. Sometimes things are nice (being fed and cuddled and warm) and sometimes things are not nice (feeding stopped, being put down). Faces and voices – or rather, images and sounds – come and go, and perhaps the first idea that recurs is that important things 'for me' happen out there, although such a fleeting notion cannot be formalised in thoughts or words. A face is associated, in due course, with the nice things happening, and the child's feelings of love and gratitude know no bounds. A face is associated with these things disappearing, forever presumably, and the child's fury is primitive and extreme. Melanie Klein called these phenomena experiences of the 'good breast' and the 'bad breast', a symbolism which put many people off from incorporating her ideas. The child lives in what Brown,[12] with greater artistry, called 'a world peopled by gods and devils'. The child experiences the first elementary sensations of love and rage in connection with this growing world around him in which he is helpless, and on which he is passively dependent. Klein called this the paranoid position in emotional development. But a most important stage is yet to come, when the child, now that his nervous system has matured a little and time has passed – he is becoming experienced – learns that the object of his hatred and the object of his love are *one and the same person*. This is an extraordinary discovery to cope with (god and devil one!) and the primitive feelings associated with this are said by Klein to form the roots of guilt and depression at what hatred he has had for the person who was so good to him, and a colossal challenge to trust, having loved his persecutor. Totally opposed feelings (ambivalence) and the pain of resolving ambivalence, have their beginnings here.

What is also important in conceptualising child development is not that these exciting adventures happened to us long ago and are now laid to rest, but were powerful enough to remain latent within us. In a stressful situation adults, like children, do tend to resort rapidly to classifying everyone into good and bad, friend and enemy. There are probably powerful evolutionary reasons why we should be able to do this, even if it can be socially very damaging. Under threat people do become 'paranoid'. This notion is compatible, also, with the impression that the capacity to become depressed, to tolerate ambiguity, to see both sides to the question, are characteristics of the mature personality.

The point about Freudian theory[34, 96, 106] is not that it is more true nor less than Kleinian theory. It makes less exciting reading than the Kleinian odyssey, but it is not incompatible with it. If Kleinian theory provides a model for the first strong feelings in a first interpersonal relationship, Freudian theory, or aspects of it, suggests that these powerful instinctive feelings derive from the dawning consciousness of a number of primitive sensations to do with basic physiological functioning: ingestion, excretion and basic life 'drive'.

Freudian theory also embodies the notion of an unfolding sequence dependent on biological development, with successive oral, anal and genital stages. The approach of Piaget[71,72,73] relates intellectual capacities such as reasoning, judgement, imagery and the capacity for symbolic thinking to the development of the brain, and provides a link between emotional and intellectual growth.

With attachment theory[8,9,10,11] there is a further link between biological, social, emotional and intellectual functioning. It proposes (i) that fundamental to survival is the capacity of the developing individual to form an internal working picture or model of his environment, so that he may explore it adequately and safely; and that equally vital for the human infant (ii) he must keep close to his parent until he is mature enough to carry out such exploration alone.

A small child near his mother in the park is a good illustration of this: up to a point feeling confident enough in the whereabouts of his mother to wander off; turning to check where he and she are; toddling away again; then hurrying back until he feels safe again and making sure he is noticed, all the time balancing his inner image of 'managing' (and the feeling of confidence that goes with it) against the proximity of his mother in reality, and how relaxed and encouraging *she* seems to be. Children watch their parents' faces like hawks. In evolutionary terms it makes sense that they should, to check whether the parent sees danger, since the parent knows what's safe and what isn't. Facial signalling between mother and baby is elaborate and important. (For an illustration of a little regression under stress, watch aircraft passengers' gaze if something alarming happens: all eyes are fixed on the faces of the cabin crew, watching for alarm signals.) According to attachment theory a sensitive, self-regulating servo-mechanism operates between child and 'caretaker', the process subserving emotional maturation. Fig. 5 illustrates it at its simplest. The child has an inborn tendency to elicit care-giving and protective behaviour from the parent. He also has an inborn tendency to explore his environment, but cannot do this (and indeed should not) unless it is safe to do so, which depends on what he sees in his environment but also on what his parent considers safe. Thus the child can explore (E), or keep closely attached to the parent (A), but can't do both. (A child can't go confidently off with his friends *and* cling to his mother's skirts or jeans.) Skilful caretaking, or parenting behaviour (C), which the child ultimately learns to trust, gets the balance right, encouraging exploration which the child can manage, responding efficiently but not excessively (over-protectively) when the child needs reassurance.

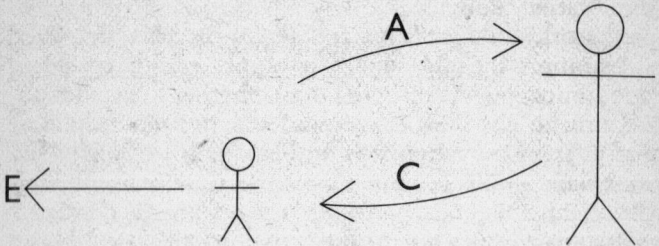

Fig. 5 Attachment behaviour – a simple model.

The important point to grasp is that this is a sensitive dynamic system operating constantly, sometimes obviously, sometimes subtly, always (with skilled parenting) achieving maximum independence for the child's age and situation. The skilled parent's glance across a room can stop a responsive child about to begin a dirty story in its tracks. Learning to explore includes learning whom not to tell rude words to. The unskilled parents and the unresponsive child, their mutual monitoring systems long abandoned as useless, may resort to mutual physical violence and still not achieve trust and control.

A further component of attachment theory is that as the system works in the real world between child and parents, he gradually builds up an inner image, a combination of memory and feeling about what was all right last time, that is the first seed of trust. Memory, feeling, the real world and its risks and opportunities, and the response of the parents carefully balanced between care and encouragement, build up a sense of confidence and competence in the child. Two ways in which it can go wrong, because of problems in the child, parent, or both, are: the child grows up fearless, promiscuous, too ready to take risks; or fearful, clinging, anxious only for safety. In a primary school on the first day you can see children who dash straight into the new classroom, fiddling with things, looking for someone to punch, and children hanging on to their tearful mothers, gazing at their faces. Teachers, it has been shown, are skilled predictors of future conduct disorder; perhaps they spot such things early.

Winnicott talked in similar terms about play.[112] Play, for a child, is an absorbing adventure full of risks, and a way of rehearsing creative and social skills. To play (and many disturbed children and adolescents cannot play) the child must feel both stimulated and safe, and the skilful parent can set the scene and handle the child to enable play to happen. In development, as in education and in psychotherapy, exploration is not only exploring the park or the playground, but experimenting, making new friends, exploring emotions and new relationships; playing new games, playing with ideas.

Many theories of development focus on childhood, and especially the young child. Erikson's theories go further and follow development into maturity, old age and death.[29,30] The characteristic feature of Erikson's theories is the concept of a series of challenges or tasks different at different times of life because of developing qualities of the individual and because of what is expected of him in his cultural setting at any particular time. The theory thus straddles psychoanalytic and anthropological thinking. At successive stages the individual has to resolve a personal 'crisis' in order to proceed effectively with emotional development. The first task is: to trust or not to trust, and later to act or not to act; to love or not to love; to make or not to make; to give or not to give; and finally, to be able to *give up* without despair. The sequence is of course far more elaborate than this brief sketch can convey. Each stage grows out of the one before, and depends in part on the previous stage being adequately negotiated; it is not a succession of isolated challenges, like hurdles.

In adolescence, the physical, intellectual and emotional equipment acquired and developed so far, and the social skills learned and social opportunities available, are put to the test again. Blos[6] has described this as a second stage of accepting and asserting individuality ('individuation'). In a maturational process consistent with the theme of attachment theory, the child is able to become independent of his parents because, if adequately cared for, he has built up within himself a sustaining, confidence-giving representation of them. Having his own 'supplies' within, he can explore independently. In adolescence, however, he must largely give this up, and find a sustaining set of new relationships in other people outside the family. This disengagement involves abandoning a bit of himself as he lets go of the close and dependent ties of childhood. According to Winnicott adolescence involves another dramatic move too; contained inevitably in the notion of independence of the parental generation is the idea of *doing without them* and the fantasy of *doing away with them*. The adolescent, representing the next generation, *will* take over, and while preparing to do so needs adults who will take responsibility and stand their ground until the younger generation can take charge and do things their own way. It seems a lot to ask; Winnicott says: 'where there is the challenge of the growing boy or girl, there let an adult meet the challenge. And it will not necessarily be nice.'[113]

Rutter's survey showed that adolescents, superficially, seem not in fact particularly rebellious.[84] Certainly large numbers of young people, perhaps the majority, appear to grow up fond of their parents and tending to share many of their views and attitudes, and this may be a credit to the skill of many parents and the more stable aspects of our culture. But it would be peculiarly unlike most aspects of human feeling, and quite out of keeping with the rest of biology, if the steady state of the more or less contented adolescent as revealed by social surveys was not determined by the interplay of forces acting in different directions, as in a parallelogram of forces, and some understanding of these forces is gained through psychodynamic theory. As already mentioned, in times and places where things do go wrong and adults abdicate from their responsibilities, young people show their destructive side and are willing to take over, wreck the joint and help man the barricades and the firing squads. History, as Berlin has pointed out, is the story of patricide.

Psychodynamic theories in perspective

The above is no more than an outline sketch of the psychodynamic approach to understanding emotional development, with Piaget slipped in since his contribution links emotional and intellectual development. The danger of psychodynamic theory is that it can be interesting and seductive and become an absorbing intellectual exercise. It says something about the development of fantasies and feelings that can be described in no other way but it must not be forgotten that such theory must take its place alongside established facts about cognitive and physical development and the facts of social life too.

Within these limitations, what contribution does the above sketch make? The work of family and social theorists tells us something about the fears and fantasies people have about a forthcoming child. Klein gives us a way of conceptualising the earliest dawning of individual feelings and ideas about what is going on 'outside', while Freudian theory proposes ways in which our physiological and anatomical functioning provide the fuel and heat and steam for this development. Taken together, psychodynamic, social and behavioural studies of babies and mothers and the rest of the family, of how adults and babies interact, and the effects of various forms of disadvantage, show how child development then takes off in a particular fashion and direction, the subsequent journey strongly influenced (but not entirely irreversibly) by what's on board.

The approaches of Bowlby, Winnicott and Erikson tell us something about early social behaviour, and how the child forms relationships with other people, incorporating strengths from the experience, so that he can deal with future experiences and gain from them too. Thus there is a progressive sequence of experience, the acquisition of skills and capacities, and experimenting with further experiences, that underlie emotional and social maturation. Finally, with all these acquired attributes and vulnerabilities aboard, the adolescent is launched into adult life, brings up children and begins to make his contribution in big ways or small to shaping the adult world. It is, after all, our children who will fix our pensions and run the geriatric services.

Do psychodynamic theories help?

In deciding what to make of psychodynamic theories of development the newcomer to the field must be as wary of those who take a 'one-theory one-therapy' line as of the unimaginative and quasi-scientific who totally dismiss the psychodynamic approach because they cannot understand it. Psychodynamic theory is a way of trying to describe and make sense of central aspects of human life and development for which there is no other language, and there is nothing particularly admirable nor scientific to refuse to have anything to do with subjective feelings and fantasies because they cannot be looked at under a microscope or measured. Psychodynamic theory is as significant a commentary on human life as are the best novels and poetry, i.e. considerably so, and is based on a number of quite different theoretical approaches.[12, 106]

It has also been a necessary stage in the development of psychological thinking, and although those who attack it point to dusty old tomes (and dusty old professionals) and say it hasn't advanced since the 1930s, in fact the key psychodynamic attitude, that not all feelings can be put into words or remembered but may still affect our behaviour, has led to important practical ways of working with disturbed children, for example in art therapy, play therapy, drama therapy, family therapy, and, of particular importance, in illuminating the relationships that develop between professional workers and their colleagues as well as their patients.

Unfortunately the psychodynamicists have let the rest of us down in a) the tendency among the less skilled majority to swallow a particular school of thought, hook, line and sinker in an uncritical fashion; b) the illusion that the child (or family) psyche can somehow float in mid-air unaccompanied by a physical body and social setting which may powerfully influence what is going on – as described earlier in this chapter; and c) by not seeing that even if their therapy *is* an art, goals can still be set and elementary research carried out on whether treatment goals can be achieved. However, it is not too late, and psychoanalytic and biological thinking are coming together in a number of interesting ways, e.g. in ethological thinking[46, 49] and in studies of attachment behaviour. The psychodynamic approach will survive its detractors, and their theories too.

Understanding abnormality

All this may seem complicated and at first sight makes the assessment of the situation of a child in difficulties seem rather daunting. In fact thinking along a number of different dimensions in this way does not require the mind of a chess master. A competent mechanic diagnosing a car breakdown considers: how old is the car? what sort of pedigree does it have and what was that year's model like? how might this particular driver have used or abused it? is there petrol in the tank? what's the weather like? if the breakdown is at the top of a hill how heavily loaded is the car? does it look well cared for? is there water in the radiator? and so on. These are simple points, but represent quite different aspects of the approach to a problem.

The problem for child psychiatry (and perhaps adult psychiatry too) is that the desire to help, and the difficulties that get in the way, can lead to professionals jumping in with whatever cluster of theories seem most attractive and with which the clinical worker feels most at home. Just because the child is taken to a psychiatrist, psychologist or social worker whose personal predilection is for, say, individual psychotherapy, or family therapy, or radical social work, does not mean that is necessarily the most helpful way of conceptualising that particular child's difficulties.

Nevertheless we cannot be totally objective. However broad a view we think we take of the total scene, planning a useful response requires focusing on particular areas, giving some more weight and more priority than others, and personal comfort and preference is bound to intrude. The attempt to take a balanced view is worth making, however, although it can be unattractive to the committed and enthusiastic 'monotherapist' who tends to expect all problems (at least the interesting ones) to fit in with his or her preferred way of working. This can be fun but is tough on the clientele. At least the attempt should be made to understand things from more than one point of view. The professional is then at least in a position to bring in an alternative source of help if the needs of the case do not match his or her own skills and preferences. The diagnostic process is discussed further in chapter 5. Here we will look briefly at how during some stage in a child's development, the idea may emerge that something is 'wrong'.

Concepts of normality and abnormality

There are three issues here;

1 Biological norms.
2 The location of the problem.
3 The attribution of disorder.

1 Biological norms

These are part of the acquired knowledge of parents and professionals, whether the facts are embodied in the culture, in technical publications, or in the useful and more widely readable books on child and adolescent development. These developmental milestones cannot be summarised here without giving a distorted, mechanistic impression. Different young people mature at different rates and in different styles, and what matters is not the obsessive matching of a child's development to a chart in a text book but that parents should be educated in child development and, where in doubt, should have ready access to friendly and informal sources of good advice. Adolescents and new parents should be helped to learn about children first by their own parents, in schools, and later by the doctors and nurses to whom they go for obstetric care. It goes without saying that such teaching needs to be informed; a good deal of rubbish about child development is still perpetuated by professionals and laymen alike.

2 The location of the problem

This is a particularly difficult and controversial subject. Much of this book is concerned with identifying the focus of the problem, which often involves a number of people, as was described in chapter 2. As much damage has been done by falsely attributing the origins of disorder to the family or parents (as in some now obsolete theories e.g. of schizophrenia and autism) as has been done by playing down the contribution family or social factors make to originating and maintaining various forms of disorder and disability.

It is important to distinguish ideas about various possible *causes* of disorder from methods of *providing help*. Thus the origin of a child's mental retardation may be entirely organic, yet the problem may well be made worse and sustained by a faulty educational approach, and distress and frustration caused all round by misplaced parental guilt and anxiety. One problem may be in a sense 'in the child's brain', and perhaps untreatable, and yet a wider view of the total difficulties leads to practical and helpful work with the child's family and the local education department.

Another aspect of the location of disorder is the way in which problems, beginning externally, come to be more and more part of the developing child's personality. For example, the way in which a family operates may clearly and openly be undermining a child's confidence and, for example, preventing him going to school without considerable anxiety. If this is clear to the professional worker, he may be able to help the parents, or the family as a whole, and reverse this anxiety-making pattern of behaviour. A mother conveying her own anxiety about school on parting with the child in the morning, and perhaps feeling insufficiently understood or supported by her husband, may be unwittingly making the child more and more nervous about school while desperately trying to persuade him that going to school is fun. At this stage, helping the family can help the child. As time passes and the child develops, the family's 'teaching' can become a self-perpetuating fearfulness *within* the child and no longer dependent on what the family as a whole is now doing. The problem may then be seen as 'in' the child and management modified accordingly, e.g. by taking an individual approach to the boy or girl as well as, or instead of, working with the rest of the family.

3 The attribution of disorder

This is the point at which referral to a psychiatrist is considered and initiated and is discussed further in chapter 8. Considering that psychiatric disorder is so ill-defined for the majority of patients who come psychiatrists' way, and that for many people it is as much a social judgement as an illness, it is surprising that the process of becoming a patient does not receive more attention in clinical circles. By and large, 'the patient' is he or she who turns up. As mentioned elsewhere, Bruggen's approach[13, 14] is an exception. (See p. 84)

Whatever our concepts of disorder, attention is drawn to something being wrong in a limited number of ways: *distress*, *disability*, worry about *symptoms*, or *complaints about behaviour*.

(a) The boy or girl may complain of feeling *distress*; feeling bad, sad, worried, muddled.

(b) The boy or girl, or an adult on their behalf, may report that there is a *disability* in its broadest sense: something someone thinks the child or adolescent ought to be able to do, but can't: read, hear, concentrate, control his or her bladder, make friends.

(c) Parents or professionals, or sometimes an older child, may report what they think are *symptoms and signs of disorder*, whether distress or disability are present or not. An unusual perceptual experience, a change in weight, odd behaviour, for example.

(d) Finally, adults may complain about *undesirable*

behaviour whether or not it seems to distress or handicap the boy or girl, usually after the failure of whatever checks and sanctions the adults concerned have been using.

One or more of these four modes of presentation will always be there, but they may not be obvious. Sometimes children and their parents arrive at child guidance clinics because they have been 'sent', and have only a vague idea as to why they are there. Perhaps the child has been difficult in the classroom, and his mother has been told to 'Take him to the clinic' and sent a slip with the appointment on it. Sometimes parents tell the child he's going to 'see the doctor' only on the morning of the appointment 'to save him worrying'. (A mother once bounded across the waiting room as I looked in, to bar my way and warn me that her daughter was 'only expecting an X-ray'.)

A more sophisticated and troublesome sort of referral, full of muddle, occurs when a case conference is held involving, say, a particularly awkward adolescent, distraught parents, child psychiatric team, local authority social worker, education welfare officer, head teacher, deputy head teacher, community physician, school doctor, probation officer and sometimes the family lawyer, backed up perhaps by the local Member of Parliament; they have met and decided that the child should be seen by another psychiatrist, usually with a view to admission to hospital. Some of them arrive on the day of the appointment (although the young person in question may have disappeared for the day), preceded and accompanied by piles of reports and letters confirming that this worker is at his wits' end, that the teacher will not have the girl back in the school until she is 'cured', and so forth, and everyone (except the girl) with a very great deal to say. At such times sorting out distress, disability, symptoms and complaints from each other, and from the background of anxiety and confusion, can be the first step in clarifying the occasion and its purpose. This is discussed further in chapter 4.

Sorting out what has gone wrong requires diagnosis, not of the child alone but of the total circumstances, without falling into the assumption that because the child has been referred there is probably something wrong with him.

Assessing the network of biological, psychological and social factors and how they interact with each other, and deciding how much weight to give to each, is of course a difficult exercise, but the theory and practice of this approach is no more elaborate than many a universal theory of psychology or sociology designed to explain everything.

When a child is in difficulties, problems are quite often multiple[79, 86] with for example learning problems, developmental difficulties, family and social problems and unhelpful extremes of parental handling (e.g. negligence or punitiveness) tending to co-exist. This does not make these factors the 'cause of the illness'. There may be emotional disorder or something like emotional disorder, and there may be factors causing it or sustaining it. Very likely there are other problems too, that require help if help is wanted for them. The professional, and especially the psychiatrist, has to take care that he distinguishes disorder, which he has some claim to be able to recognise and offer to treat, from other problems, which he may help clarify but which others may help more effectively.

How many children are psychiatrically disturbed?

The answer to this question depends on yet another factor: where you draw the line. Until we define psychiatry's role we can hardly begin to define its clientele. If child and adolescent psychiatrists limit their role in the way suggested later in this book, the number of

young people needing psychiatrists is smaller than if
you believe we need vast numbers of child psychiatrists
to treat mentally handicapped children and delinquents,
offer counselling in schools, run therapeutic communities and so. When it is suggested that more resources for disturbed children are needed, for example
in the Court report[25] it is most important to try to define
what exactly is needed, and whether it should be a
primarily psychiatric service (i.e. a hospital or clinic), or
something primarily educational, social or custodial and
supervisory.

With these cautionary words, it can be said that the
thoroughly conducted survey of the incidence of child
psychiatric disorders on the Isle of Wight[90] showed a
prevalence of around 5 per cent at age ten and eleven of
psychiatric disorder among over 2000 children in this age
range. Of these disorders, the majority were emotional
and conduct disorders. The more serious disorders listed
in chapter 5 such as hyperkinetic syndrome, autism and
severe phobic and obsessional states were rare or non-
existent. It is worth noting, however, that taking all
forms of chronic handicap together, including intellectual and physical handicap, 17 per cent of children
were in some degree of difficulty.

Schools, neighbourhoods and areas of the country
vary considerably in the incidence of psychiatric disorder, broadly defined, as well as in delinquency and
reading problems,[83,86] with the greater incidence of
problems found in the more disadvantaged groups of the
population. Moreover, these problems are inter-related
– for example conduct problems and reading difficulties.
They are also variably noticed by adults,[84] and the
incidence of psychiatric disorders rises in adolescence,
but once again the incidence varies with how the problem is defined. In general figures between 10–20 per
cent are given.[37,57] Probably the best range of figures to
keep in mind is that over the course of a year between
5–15 per cent of children experience handicapping psy-

chiatric (largely emotional and conduct) disorder, and that there is a rise to perhaps 15–20 per cent in adolescence.[25,37,80] However, it is important to emphasise that this is *not* to suggest that all these young people need psychiatrists, although many need special attention including professional help.

Conclusions

Throughout the twenty years or so of development from dependent infancy to independent adulthood there is a 'fallout': the abused child; the boy who can't comprehend and use language; the girl who panics when away from her parents; the child whose intellectual level leaves him unable to cope with what is expected of most of the others in his age group; the adolescent, torn between achieving independence and fearing adulthood, who tries to stop the clock by holding her weight just below that at which sexual maturation occurs, and develops anorexia nervosa; the depressed child; the fearful child and the incorrigibly naughty child. How they have come to be this way depends on the complicated interplay, over the years, of biological, psychological and social factors.

The great majority of these children in difficulties have problems with their emotional and social development and in their education and behaviour. Their number, overall, depends on how disorder is defined, which age group is being considered, and where they live, and it varies accordingly around 5–15 per cent. Most need special help of some sort. A small number need psychiatric help. How many need psychiatric help, what sort, and how it is best delivered, is the wider theme of the rest of the book.

4

Child Psychiatry I: Disorders, Diagnosis and the Referral Process

Introduction: the story so far

Many things can go wrong in a child's life leaving him worried, miserable, unable to cope with some aspect of home or school life, or the object of complaint or concern. Up to a point such variations in mood, behaviour and performance are regarded as within the province of the child's parents or teachers; they try to understand the boy or girl, try different approaches, perhaps seek some advice from a friend, relative or book.

To this extent it may be acknowledged that the problem is shared. If a teacher has a general approach to discipline which is his own style, and which works for most children, but finds he has to be firmer with a particular boy or girl, then he does not think there is something 'wrong' with the child but rather that he, the teacher, had not at first taken the right approach. He needs to change as much as the child.

Exactly the same applies to a child's problem in learning. Up to a point, the teacher uses different aspects of his repertoire of skills to help different children achieve various goals. But there comes a point where the effort, skill and indeed time required to deal with a child's behaviour or ability to learn, perhaps with small return for the trouble taken, marks the child out as different from most.

In what way is he different? A child who, for example, cannot learn does not necessarily have a learning problem as such. Perhaps the first thing a teacher might wonder about a child found to be in difficulties is whether he is worried about something at school or at home. He or she might turn out to have a hearing defect or need glasses.

Failure to cope with a child's educational, emotional or behavioural problems on the part of the adults normally involved with him – parents and teachers – is the beginning of a move towards getting the help of specialists: people with the training, but also provided with the time and the setting, to concentrate on the special difficulty. It may invoke simply advice, or extra sessions of special help, or a move to a completely different setting. The girl in chapter 2 ended up in a highly specialised setting, for example, waiting in a hospital casualty department for someone willing to take over the task of *holding her still*.

This move towards the specialist involves two assumptions: (i) that the present people cannot provide what the boy or girl needs for their mood, behaviour or education; (ii) that in some way the boy or girl is disordered – not working properly. These parallel strands wind around each other like a double helix. *Of course* a particular girl is quite unmanageable *because* her family is breaking up, her father a violent alcoholic and her mother depressed, and she is getting worse *because* in the classroom she is smelly and unpopular and the teacher cannot manage her. The girl isn't right and the setting isn't right, and each is making the other worse.

But the move towards the specialist setting has contained within it the notion that the right setting has now been found, and as the girl moves into it she is regarded as the more abnormal for being there. Home and classroom are no longer part of her problem. She and her problem are now tidily put away into the special setting, such as the 'maladjusted' boarding school or the children's home. It is not that this step is wrong; it is simply that it is important to appreciate what is going on, namely a subtle but significant change in her personal status. That child 'has' appendicitis. This child 'is' maladjusted.

It is not, after all, *totally* different from the child with appendicitis going into hospital. One strand of the two still applies: the parents can no more manage the inflamed appendix than the school can manage the awkward girl. But the other strand is different, in that (for argument's sake) the appendix is demonstrably infected and inflamed and is rightly in hospital and to be cut out, while the girl's problem behaviour is not entirely carried around inside her, but partly dependent on the adults around her and how they look after her.

Meanwhile, for the purposes of this chapter, the issue is not what to do, but what's wrong; and diagnosis means *knowing thoroughly*; '*perceiving through*'.

At this point I would like to pre-empt an observation that comes later, and suggest that in child and adolescent psychiatry diagnosis has two central aims:

1 *Identifying and describing clinical psychiatric disorder, if any;*
2 *Making a broader diagnostic formulation of what factors, biological, social and psychological, have conspired to bring the child to the psychiatrist, whether or not psychiatric disorder is among them.*

The process of making a diagnosis is very close to the heart of the much-maligned 'medical model', and like medicine itself is frequently and erroneously believed to be a fundamentally physically-orientated preoccupation. Diagnosis means knowing, or finding out, what is wrong, and among the fundamentals of various ancient trades and crafts, the essence of the medical approach has always been to diagnose what is wrong. Treatment, physical or otherwise, has never been a strong point.

The craftsman makes something for his customer; the

teacher instructs his pupil; the lawyer speaks on his behalf; the policeman enforces limits on behaviour; the trader obtains and sells things. The physician establishes if something is 'wrong' with someone, and tries to find ways of putting it right by treatment or 'therapy'. The ever-hopeful researching and developing of treatment techniques has always been a major part of medical industry, with adequate understanding of disorders lagging quite some way behind optimistic empirical efforts. When psychologists, social workers or psycho-therapists use the concept of something being 'wrong' with their clients as individuals, and needing their own particular brand of therapy (be it behaviour therapy or drama therapy or psychotherapy or whatever), they are using the medical model, although it may grieve them to know this.

Diagnosis smacks of labelling and pigeon-holing. Rutter has pointed out that it is the disorder that is classified, not the child.[78] If a number of characteristics of a child are seen in other children, tend to take a particular course, are associated with certain other circumstances in their background and especially if this cluster of phenomena sometimes responds to a par-ticular sort of help, it seems reasonable (to doctors, because that is how we are trained) to give that particular cluster of phenomena and circumstances a name. Then we can talk to other people who are trying to help that particular problem in the knowledge that we are prob-ably talking about the same thing.

Schizophrenia, for example, is a diagnosis that many psychiatrists will agree about if they use certain inter-national criteria for the disorder.[116] This is an important start, even if the causes, contributing factors and treat-ment of the schizophrenic illnesses remain uncertain.

The hyperkinetic syndrome is a good example of a disorder which appears to be common in the United States and rare in the United Kingdom,[16,90] a phenom-enon almost certainly due to different sorts of doctors rather than different sorts of children.

Rutter and his colleagues working with the World Health Organisation, have developed a scheme for the classification of children's disorders based as far as possible on the grouping together under headings of reasonably objective observations.[88, 89] The scheme prejudges neither cause nor treatment but is an attempt to get agreement over the description of what is going on: the diagnosis.

The system puts observations under five headings, each representing quite different dimensions, or axes, of the child's life.

Axis 1: Clinical psychiatric syndrome
Axis 2: Developmental disorders
Axis 3: Intellectual level
Axis 4: Physical health and ability
Axis 5: Psychosocial situation

Clinical psychiatric syndrome

This is the traditional medical diagnosis: a term for a cluster of symptoms (things reported, like bed wetting) and signs (things observed by the clinician, like poor attention span). The word 'syndrome' means a cluster of symptoms and signs; the psychiatric syndromes of childhood are discussed later.

Developmental disorder

The psychiatric disorders are based on a multiplicity of symptoms and signs, peculiarities in mood and thinking and behaviour. But some disorders seem more readily understood in terms of delay in the acquisition of skills which normally come with increasing growth and maturation. Thus the ability to use speech or read may present unusual difficulties in a particular child's case, and be quite handicapping. Again this would say nothing about the child's intelligence or mental health, either or both of which may be normal. These developmental delays are specific in the sense that the disability is out of proportion to the child's general level of ability, as in specific reading retardation (dyslexia).

Intellectual level

Intelligence, based on intelligence tests, is an entirely artificial but useful measure of an individual's capacity for reasoning, just as a column of mercury in a glass tube is an artificial but useful measure of an individual's heat. The intelligence quotient (IQ) expresses how successful a child is compared with others in a similar age-range doing the same tests. The widely used test in this country is the *WISC* (Wechsler Intelligence Scale for Children) but there are others which the psychologist selects for different purposes as any other diagnostician selects the right tool for the job. But in comparing one child with another intellectually, account has to be taken of the sorts of test used, just as one cannot compare Centigrade temperature with Fahrenheit without allowing for the different scales. The normal range of intelligence is the wide range within which most children (97 per cent) operate – 70–140, with the greatest number closest to the mean, 100. It is *normal* to have an intelligence of 75 and of 135, but they will be two very different children.

It is not statistically normal to have an intellectual level less than 70, nor greater than 140, but that does not mean disorder (one of the syndromes) is present. A child may be mildly, moderately, or severely intellectually retarded (or mentally handicapped) but even though the effect of the low intellectual level can be a problem, perhaps a major one, the description of the child under this heading says nothing about any other axis.

Physical health and ability

A boy or girl may be physically fit or a physical disorder or defect, major or minor may be present: epilepsy, defective vision, hearing impairment, diabetes mellitus, abnormality of stature, meningitis, asthma, and so on. This is important as a component of the child's life, whatever its bearing on the presenting problem. A child's epilepsy may or may not have any direct physical bearing on his mood and behaviour at school; the fact that his parents are extremely anxious and protective towards him may. Regardless of possible use in a total diagnosis of the child in his situation, or in plans for treatment, the fact of his health is recorded.

Psychosocial situation

This is an interesting and important category, straddling a whole range of concepts that have variously been called in to account for or describe disorder and disadvantage. The scheme[89] lists sixteen (e.g. inadequate linguistic stimulation; inconsistent handling; excess or lack of discipline; neglect; family breakdown; poverty; persecution; social crisis; natural disaster; and others) and its framework has room for eighty-three more categories as yet unformulated.

A child could be presented to a child psychiatric team as disordered, but the only diagnosis possible might come in this last category, e.g. trouble in the family, or the neighbourhood; but no mental illness, intellectual problem, developmental disorder or abnormality of physical health.

Relationship between diagnosis and services: an example

The use of this scheme has a direct link with the theme of the proper use and development of services for children. An extreme example, and one that unhappily will be familiar to many, is that of the child with multiple and chronic problems. One may see perplexed and profoundly worried parents of adolescents with, for example, brain damage and autism, whose experience is of their child moving from specialist to specialist, school to school, and home to home over the years, never feeling settled anywhere, and always with a different 'diagnosis'. One doctor said the child was psychotic, another that he was autistic, another that he was mentally handicapped, another that he was epileptic, another that he was in the wrong sort of school, or that the family home wasn't the best place for him. The parents don't know what to make of all these very different opinions; in fact they are all accurate descriptions of the child's multiple problems. He may well be autistic (a category of psychosis, Axis 1), intellectually retarded (Axis 3), but with no specific developmental delay (Axis 2), suffer from temporal lobe epilepsy (Axis 4) and his most pressing problem is that the sort of home and school that can contain him for sufficiently long to help his social training and education has yet to be found. Probably most of the ten to twenty specialists who successively offer advice in such cases, over the years, are aware of other aspects of the child's complex problems.

Conceivably it would have helped if, early on, someone had said:

This child has the beginnings of a chronic problem for which there is no cure, and he needs a long-term home and school with the confidence and strength to contain him long enough for him to learn something, including normal behaviour; advice will be needed on the child's psychiatric state and epilepsy (such advice being available from nearby clinics to all under the National Health Service, whether in a residential institution or not), and the parents will need support and help over the years to face the disappointment of their child's problem.

Instead, characteristically, such a family will have been to psychoanalytically-orientated teachers, therapeutic communities, neurologists, paediatricians, psychiatrists and psychologists in the NHS and private practice, community physicians, school doctors, social workers, children's hospitals, and all sorts of psychiatric and mental handicap hospitals, with little if any sustained help or sense of being helped.

This is not to say that the above 'prescription' could easily be put into practice. But until the prescription and other prescriptions are issued with reasonable consistency, the necessary facilities will not even be thought of, let alone established. And there are many less dramatic examples of the same sort of problem: the child's difficulty seen first one way, then another, then another, then back to the first again, driven more by whoever (child, family, or specialist) is feeling the most anxious that day, rather than planned rationally according to the child's and family's total needs.

Some terminological problems: 'mental illness', 'emotional disturbance', etc.

This particular nettle had better be grasped. These terms have no very precise meanings, and are used partly for variety but partly to imply differing degrees of severity.

There are many variations in usage. What matters finally, is a clear statement of the problem in each child's case rather than which of these particular headings it is allotted. *Problems* are problems, before one has decided whether they are illnesses or disorders or anything else.

Emotional disorder and illness
This term tends to refer to mild to moderate abnormalities in mood, for example, when a child has periods

of misery or fearlessness or bad temper, abnormal in degree or persistence, whatever the cause.

I reserve the term *illness* for the more severe, entrenched problems which seem to be largely self-perpetuating within the boy or girl, and suggestive of a disease process, such as schizophrenia or the more severe forms of depression with physiological symptoms such as loss of weight and sleep. If it is an illness, I tend to link to it the term *psychiatric*, or its synonym *mental*.

Disturbance and personality disorder

This is a conveniently ambiguous term, since a child may be disturbed from within or without.

The term *personality disorder* is widely used in adult psychiatry. I never apply it to children or adolescents because their personalities are still in the process of developing; for the same reason one cannot speak of children or adolescents having *established* patterns of sexual preferences, whether regarded as abnormal or not. However, if a boy or girl is beginning to show persisting traits or problems in their attitudes and behaviour, independent of any illness, it is reasonable to refer to this as problematic *(or abnormal) personality development*. This term carries with it implications of further growth and change, and is sufficiently different to justify the distinction from the term personality disorder with its intimations of permanence.

Delinquency

This is a legal term, not a clinical one. Most delinquents are not disordered. However, if a child with a conduct (or any other) disorder breaks the law, he is then a delinquent too.

The psychiatric syndromes of childhood

A classification scheme of the psychiatric syndromes is set out below, and, it will be remembered, constitutes only one of the five dimensions in which each child's problems are considered.

The syndromes represent clinical findings – symptoms and signs. Some problems are so common that they acquire some of the connotations of a syndrome themselves, but in fact they are not. Thus *school refusal*, in a particular child's case, may in the event turn out to be properly categorised as phobic anxiety, depression or family disturbance. *Attempted suicide* may be carried out by a child whose problems are best stated as depression, conduct disorder, or again as a family or social problem.

The syndromes listed below will only be outlined here: what follows is essentially a glossary. Detail would distract from the book's theme, and there are excellent books available which describe these disorders in more depth.[2,81,85] This further reading is recommended because what follows is necessarily brief and dogmatic.

Before proceeding with the list of disorders, it is worth emphasising another reason for having such categories. It is characteristic of the proponents of 'universal theories', explanations of human problems in unitary psychological or sociological terms, to denigrate medical-type diagnoses as inhuman and even oppressive. Unfortunately it is also characteristic of those who think in such terms, while denying the existence of psychiatric illness, to tend to label all comers in an allegedly more humanistic style: 'mixed up', oppressed, alienated, invalidated, unfulfilled or whatever. The implications for any community of this insidious assumption of helplessness in the face of hypothetical pressures from within or without is beyond the scope of this book. But for psychiatry to maintain and improve its integrity

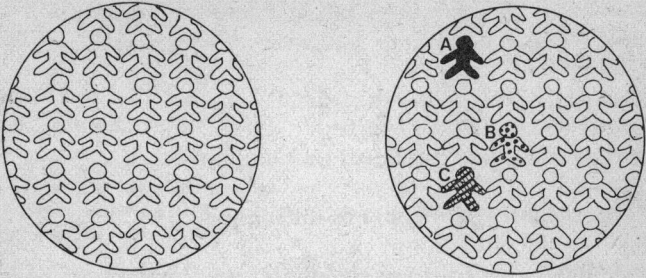

Fig. 6 Universal theory versus clinical category.

it is important for it to develop the idea of disorders which it is its business and skill to pick out from those referred, which means being prepared to make no clinical diagnosis in the cases where there are no clinical symptoms and signs, *whatever* problem that individual is experiencing or presenting to the community. The former system could find a label for *everyone* in sociological, behavioural or psychoanalytical lines, although for the moment this may not matter too much. The clinical diagnostic system picks out those who show disorder in clinical terms.

Classification Scheme

Emotional disorders: persisting, abnormal and handicapping mood states
Depression, misery, unhappiness predominating
Sensitivity, shyness and social withdrawal; elective mutism
Phobic, obsessional, hypochondriacal and hysterical states of childhood

Conduct disorders: persisting, abnormal and problematic behaviour patterns causing social disapproval
Unsocialised conduct disorder
Socialised conduct disorder
Mixed disorder of conduct and emotions

Hyperkinetic syndrome of childhood

Psychotic disorders of childhood (i.e. beginning before puberty)
Infantile autism (Kanner's syndrome)
Disintegrative psychosis
Childhood schizophrenia

Adult-type psychotic and other disorders
Schizophrenia
Depressive and manic depressive illness
Neurotic depression
Drug and alcoholic psychoses
Drug and alochol dependence
Non-dependent abuse of drugs
Transient organic psychotic disturbances
Depersonalisation syndrome

Chronic organic psychotic disorders

Acute reactions to stress, and less transient adjustment reactions

Other syndromes
Stammering and stuttering
Anorexia nervosa
Other disorders of eating
Tics
Sleep disorders
Enuresis (involuntary wetting)
Encopresis (soiling)

Emotional disorders, conduct disorders and 'mixed' emotional and conduct disorders[41,117]

Emotional disorders, which with *conduct disorders* constitute by far the most common problems of childhood referred to psychiatrists, are also the least well differentiated, and are very commonly practically impossible to separate from the context in which they occur. A child's misery, fearfulness or misbehaviour, even when to some extent self-perpetuating, is very often maintained by how other people in his or her life are behaving. Similarly *conduct disorder*, defined as abnormal behaviour causing social disapproval, is clearly heavily dependent on the rules and attitudes of the community in which it occurs. It is fashionable to hold that if a Western culture disapproves of certain behaviour, the culture is wrong, not the individual. Certainly the difference between the 'disordered' on the one hand and the dissident on the other is a matter over which psychiatry needs to take very great care indeed. However, children categorised as being conduct disordered are not confident young radicals, but usually unhappy children from disturbed families, they frequently have educational and specific reading problems, and the outlook for them with or without treatment, tends to be poor. Many grow up to have major personality, social and family problems. Most children with emotional problems, however, tend to get better, although social and educational damage can be done along the way.

'Mixed' disorders is the classification for children with both conduct problems and emotional problems. 'Unsocialised' conduct disorder refers to solitary stealing, disobedience, aggressiveness and other unpopular behaviour which the child initiates alone. 'Socialised' conduct disorder refers to group behaviour of this sort. Conduct disorder is commoner in boys, but emotional disorders occur about equally in both sexes.

Emotional disorders characteristic of younger children tend to be less clearly differentiated. A child will often be miserable, or frequently fearful. He or she may have tummy-aches, be phobic of certain situations or objects, and have disabling comforting or repetitive habits. In older childhood, and particularly adolescents, the child's greater maturity, self-expression and more advanced social role together give these disorders more of the quality of adult-type neurotic conditions. Whether they are different in any other sense is hard to say.

Other adult-type problems occur in childhood too, and the possibility of their existence is kept in mind in any age group. Physical illness, whether or not of the central nervous system, the effects of toxic substances administered by the child or by adults (alcohol, glue solvents, amphetamines, barbiturates, heroin, Valium, thalidomide, lead, for example), and the rare brain degenerative disorders of young people do occur.

A puzzling problem of adolescents is the 'borderline' state, characterised by strong and mixed feelings, major social handicaps, in particular unhappy eccentricity and social withdrawal, and bizarre ideas and behaviour. There is a good deal of disagreement about this disorder and its relationship with schizophrenic-like disorders on the one hand and emotional and personality disorders on the other. It also is uncommon.

Reactions to stress

A catastrophic emotional reaction to a severe external stress needs help whether or not it is regarded as a psychiatric disorder. Major loss or social crises such as accidents, social upheaval and natural disasters are among the possible causes, and may be extremely tragic. One observation of such major losses and disasters is the resilience of children if their earlier life was stable, and if the adults looking after them through the crisis cope with their own and their children's needs and feelings reasonably competently and without chaos and panic.

Other non-psychotic syndromes of childhood and adolescence

Anorexia nervosa[22, 23, 52] is one of the best known disorders of adolescence, occurring mostly, but not entirely, in girls. Refusal to eat, serious loss of weight and amenorrhoea constitute the syndrome, and the most striking anxiety of the young person concerned appears to be a fear of gaining weight, possibly coupled with a fear of achieving physical maturity, rather than a fear of food. It appears to be becoming more common, and can be a seriously handicapping and dangerous disorder, sometimes leading to death. Obesity can be a problem in children and adolescents too.[19]

Tics[21] are involuntary and apparently purposeless movements occurring in the absence of disease of the nervous system. A rare tic disorder is Gilles de la Tourett's syndrome in which marked facial and other involuntary jerking is accompanied by involuntary noises and obscene words and sentences. The utterances, obscene or not, are both involuntary, or under very little control, and likely to upset the person to whom they are addressed; the sufferer from this grossly handicapping disorder often finds himself unable to contain remarks he knows will be particularly upsetting to the people who hear them.

The hyperkinetic syndrome of childhood[16] is of considerable interest since it is rarely diagnosed in the UK, while a few years ago it was being diagnosed in as many as 40 per cent of child guidance clinic attenders in the United States. Almost certainly this represented the mis-diagnosis (or, more politely, difference in terminology) whereby children with conduct problems were being regarded as having this syndrome. In this country it is tightly defined as a gross disturbance of behaviour with poor attention span, striking distractibility, disinhibited and impulsive behaviour, often accompanied by self-neglectful, high-risk behaviour. Parents will report that the child seems unaware of danger and will dash straight into the road. Anyone who has ever met a hyperkinetic child as here defined would not mistake it for naughtiness. The naughty child, up to a point where his naughtiness is interrupted, seems to be enjoying himself. The hyperkinetic child characteristically is all over the place, breaking up his (and other people's) things, hurriedly dropping one activity and beginning another, only to go on restlessly and not particularly happily to something else, then something else, then something else again. Some hyperkinetic children become slow and apathetic in adolescence. There is often developmental delay too, and indeed the disorder has many characteristics of a temperamental abnormality, and yet the disturbed behaviour itself is often dependent on the situation the child is in at the time.

Adult-type disorders and other syndromes. Most children with emotional problems get over them, but some become 'neurotic' in adult life. 'Neurotic' is as vague a term as 'psychotic', but includes a fairly well differentiated set of emotional problems such as *phobias* (specific fears), *obsessional-compulsive states* (thinking or behaviour the individual tries with limited success to resist, and which can become grossly handicapping) and *depressive states* which appear less severe than psychotic depression, and more related to personality difficulties and life problems. The relationship between the two extremes of depression is immensely complicated and endlessly discussed by psychiatrists.

Stammering, or *stuttering*, is a common and often transient problem in the articulation of speech, and may or may not be associated with emotional difficulties.

Enuresis[94] is a well known nuisance, usually as

nocturnal enuresis or bed wetting. By seven years 20 per cent of children still wet the bed occasionally, and by fifteen, 3 per cent do. It is associated with emotional or behavioural difficulties in only about a third of cases. Probably many cases are accounted for by the effects of greater or lesser degrees of stress (and what is stressful is of course subjective) on bladder control which is achieved variably by different children. It is unusual for a psychiatrist to be able to identify the cause of bed wetting in a particular child's case.

Encopresis[42] or faecal soiling may have a similar origin to enuresis (the effect of stress on the gradual acquisition of control) or it may have a physical cause. Thus if for some reason the passage of faeces is painful, constipation can occur, with liquid motions leaking past. Encopresis can be more elaborate in emotional and conduct disorders, when the child secretes his motions around various parts of the house.

Sleep, in children as in adults, is vulnerable to physical and emotional disorders as well as to the day's excitements. It may be disturbed (e.g. insomnia, excessive sleep, night terrors) in a variety of disorders, or in relation to none in particular.

Sexual problems[38], the *abuse of drugs and alcohol*[7, 20, 62] and other problems of life-style and behaviour occur in older children and adolescents. Sometimes an ingrained and disabling habit develops, and can be hard to break; but it is important to remember that behind the headlines about drug-taking and glue-sniffing young people with their attendant notoriety, there may be not so much a 'disorder' as a child who is being inadequately supervised, if not neglected, or who, because of some more general family problems, doesn't care what his parents think.

As mentioned earlier, such problems as *school non-attendance*,[43, 81] *child abuse, attempted suicide*[54, 92] and also *repeated running away from home* are not themselves disorders but may be evidence of disorder, which may turn out to be individual, in the family or socially determined.

Psychotic disorders in children

Psychotic disorders[97,109] are rare. Schizophrenic-like disorders and manic-depressive and depressive illnesses can begin in childhood and adolescence, usually no earlier than around puberty.

Autism,[109] also known as Kanner's syndrome, is perhaps the best known childhood psychosis and is also rare. It begins in infancy and is characterised by failure of development of the understanding and use of language, and of normal social relationships, and by stereotyped, ritualistic, non-creative activities instead of play. It is a quite different disorder from schizophrenia but many American authors have used the terms autism, childhood schizophrenia and childhood psychosis interchangeably, which is confusing. The old notion that the parents of autistic children themselves have special emotional or communication problems is not true, but they do tend to be middle class. Why they should be is a subject for dispute.[110]

Autism is not the same problem as mental retardation. About three-quarters of autistic children also have varying degrees of mental retardation, others having intelligence in the normal range, but these children do tend to have special problems in comprehension and imaginative thinking. The best outlook is for those with the highest levels of intelligence and use of language.

Clinical diagnosis and the diagnostic formulation

While the *diagnosis* is a word or two identifying a disorder, most psychiatrists find it helpful to make a *diagnostic formulation*, which is a statement, often in several sentences, of the various factors making up the problem. These include the five descriptive axes already given, plus a hypothesis about the way they may have interacted, and this can include ideas about individual psychodynamic or family dynamic factors. A note about outlook and plans for management complete this statement.

Suppose a girl has been referred as an emergency by worried parents and teachers at a school for mentally retarded youngsters. She has been behaving oddly and they feel she may be acutely psychotic and in need of admission to hospital.

The clinical diagnosis (Axis 1) may be *mixed disorder of conduct and emotions*. In addition there is *developmental abnormality of motor co-ordination* (clumsiness (Axis 2)); *mild mental retardation* (IQ 60) (Axis 3); *anoxic brain damage*, which occurred at birth (Axis 4); *school and family problems* (Axis 5).

The diagnostic formulation is: A thirteen year old girl with mild mental retardation due to long-established brain damage who has done quite well at two special schools, but the move to a third has coincided with the onset of adolescence and a marked growth spurt. The combination of her physical growth, the expression of angry feelings about her handicap, and the unfamiliar setting have led to problems in her behaviour.

The family's move from another part of the country and away from supportive relatives has made the child's anger harder to cope with, and has renewed in the parents their old feelings of guilt, anxiety and lack of confidence in professional opinion, both educational and medical. The strength of their doubts and feelings is now leading to equivalent anxieties in the teachers and doctors, who are also beginning to feel that she should be in a different school or even in hospital.

In fact there is no reason why the girl should not settle down at her new school if the teachers are offered advice and help and if the parents are helped to ventilate and discuss their uncertainties, look at ways in which they can settle down in their new neighbourhood, and discuss their misgivings with their daughter's new teachers.

Plan: The psychiatric team needs to see the girl only infrequently, but one of them will work out with the girl's teachers ways to manage her misbehaviour and assess progress, while the social worker will meet the parents fortnightly for a few months. Regular though not necessarily frequent meetings between the teachers, the psychiatric team members and the family would be a helpful way of reviewing progress and affirming that support and advice is available.

Overall aim: To see if child and family can be helped to overcome their anxieties and settle down in the new school and home, and only then to see if any reasons remain for a radical change in further plans for the girl. This may not work. The parents' doubts may be too profound. The school might turn out to be the wrong one, perhaps handling the child badly and unable to change its approach. The point is *not* to regard the parents as 'neurotic' or the school as either ideal or incapable, but to help channel strong feelings into productive directions and 'hold' the situation while a careful assessment is made of a) what the child needs, b) what the adults, parents and teachers can provide with help. It *could* emerge after all that the child needs a period in hospital. But an emergency dash from school to hospital, abandoning what has been done so far and hoping for something new with no special goals for the admission, not only undermines the girl, the school, the family and raises false hopes, but is more likely to be based on adults' anxieties than the child's true needs.

When things settled down again, it emerged that when the teachers seemed unable to cope, the girl's parents had indeed experienced once again long-standing fears, never far away, that the girl would one day end up in an awful long-stay hospital for the mentally handicapped, especially as she (and they) grew older. In their panic, they felt that at least urgent admission to a modern acute psychiatric unit for young people would be marginally 'better' and might even diagnose the cause of their child's handicap, and find a 'cure'. Again, old and sadly irrational hopes, mingled with mixed feelings about what doctors might or might not be able to do, were resurrected. They recalled their child's infancy, when a succession of doctors had raised hopes, admittedly vaguely, never fulfilled.

What did diagnosis indicate was needed?

(a) Checking the nature and extent of the girl's handicaps, emotional, intellectual and developmental, if this had not already been done elsewhere.

(b) Checking that the school was the right one, and able to do the right things for the girl's care and education, including setting limits on her misbehaviour.

(c) Helping the school to contain her in the light of her behaviour and the parents' doubts.

(d) Helping the parents sort out reasonable from unreasonable doubts for themselves, so that ultimately they could make their own decision on a better basis.

The diagnostic process in principle

Different child psychiatrists work differently, but in general they would want to know:

(a) *What is everyone involved concerned about?* What for example are the child's problems, the parents' anxieties, the teacher's complaints about the child? Who is complaining about what?

(b)   *How has the present referral come about?* What was the sequence by which a boy or girl was identified rightly or wrongly as (i) needing special help, (ii) needing a psychiatrist's help.

(c)   *What is the child's history?* In understanding a child's development we are dealing with biography – the story of his or her life. The best biographies and autobiographies begin with grandparents and great-grandparents and even the geography and the history of the time, well before the birth of their subject.

Taking an adequate history can be a lengthy process and doesn't amount to merely ticking off a list of essential questions. Many psychiatrists try to get a good outline of the child's biography at the first session, although not everyone works this way. Some psycho-therapists and family therapists are more inclined to wait and see what comes, believing that everything important will emerge in due course if the therapist is patient and encourages talk and thought around important *present* matters, and avoids the more interrogatory style of history taking.

The child's history, then, is the family history. What sort of baby did they want? What fears and fantasies and family myths were there? How was the birth? What sort of an experience was it? How did mother, father, child and the rest of the family relate to each other thereafter? A complex and developing interaction of child and mother and family, referred to in chapter 3, makes up the total story of the child's life so far.

But while carefully putting together this story, with all its inevitable gaps, exaggerations, faulty recollec-tions and indeed disagreement about what happened, the psychiatrist will also be listening and watching for two other dimensions of the tale. First, do the feelings expressed *now* throw light on how things were then? Second, what was life actually like when these events were taking place?

A psychiatrist may learn from the history that a second child was born while the first child was an awkward toddler; that the mother's father had just had the first bad coronary from which he later died; that an aunt was mentally ill; that there was a period of anxiety when an older child had some symptoms reminiscent of an illness from which a young relation had become disabled; that from time to time the child's father was drinking rather heavily and mother got depressed; that her own mother was a particularly critical woman. It may also emerge that some of these things were happening in sequence, and close together, adding up to a cumulative strain.

It is difficult to recreate what life might have actually been like eight, nine or fifteen years before; the mother's anxiety about feeling more and more inadequate and depressed and not knowing why, but fearing she might 'go like Aunt Maud' who was in and out of mental hospitals; fearing her mother's criticism, and her husband turning away from the chaotic household and to his own mother and to alcohol, and the older child, just starting school, developing tummy-aches. The younger child, tense, feeding poorly, intermittently and unpredictably left alone for long periods, sometimes cuddled by a tearful mother, sometimes smacked for crying, fed angrily. In turn the child responding erratically to his mother's moods, for example not smiling when a smile would have rewarded her, so she finds the child hard to cope with and gets angrier with herself, more despairing about her real and imagined inadequacies, and angrier with the child, who gets more anxious and less able to feed easily, smile easily, play easily or learn new things (like bladder control) easily: instead, a 'difficult' child.

It is not that such experiences 'cause' later problems. Rather they set the pattern of child-parental interaction which continues uneasily, now all right, now not all right, now vulnerable because of a move of house, now bad.

But many families have problems, the story has to make sense, although inevitably there are gaps. What has stopped the ordinary supportive and coping and learning mechanisms operating? Is the child constitutionally vulnerable, perhaps slow to learn some skills? Or have external stresses been the last straw? What needs to be done to help things on to an even keel again? What's missing, or been badly handled?

More specifically, the child's general health, patterns of eating and sleeping, capacity to play and make friends and concentrate, ability to use language and other means of self-expression, relationships with other people, reaction to discipline, separation from parents, self-control, school performance and sexual behaviour are all facets of a total developmental sequence, and need to be known.

(d) *With what predispositions might the child have been born?* Again, as part of the family story, what has been passed on in the genes? Most disorders are not directly hereditary. Schizophrenia, bed wetting or poor reading may not be handed on intact, as it were; but the son of a man who was enuretic, for example, may be a little slow to learn bladder control, and his bladder control vulnerable under stress (perhaps a stress made worse because of father's reluctance to talk about it). Exactly the same may be true of an inherited predisposition to having trouble with recognising and sequencing letters and words; inherited vulnerability (trivial or marked), and parental anxiety (trivial or marked), together may trigger a disability by adding anxiety to a learning or developmental problem.

These are not given as examples of how bed wetting or specific reading retardation usually develop, but as a guide to a *style of thinking* as a child's and family's story develop: what biological, social and psychological factors are interweaving?

(e) *What sort of environment has the child grown up in?* What was it like in earlier years? How has it been recently? But as well as the social and cultural facts, the parents' and grandparents' ethical values, beliefs and attitudes are important too. All very well for a child to be reported as 'masturbating'. So what? Does it matter? Why do the parents think it matters? What information or misinformation have they been given? And the physical environment (nutrition, pollution) is noted.

(f) *How is the child and his or her environment now?* This is partly what the child psychiatrist sees for himself, partly what he is told by the family. What are the child's thoughts and feelings and social behaviour like now? How intelligent is the child? Does he or she have specific learning problems, such as troubles in reading or language greater than to be expected from his or her level of intelligence? What about present relationships with the rest of the family, with friends, with teachers? What do other people make of the child's difficulties? What do they do to make things better or worse? As well as the child's strengths and weaknesses and potential, the strengths and weaknesses and capacity for change of the family and of the child's teachers and other significant adults is a factor too. If a child has become sexually disinhibited or developed phobic or obsessional habits, and needs a firm hand and an honest and confident approach, can the parents do it? Can the teachers do it? If not, could they do it if helped? If not, how important is it that it be done? Important enough for the child to be away from home or at another school? This clearly depends on what the people involved want too. Odd sexual behaviour, for example, may be tolerated differently, say, in a convent and in a modern school (perhaps better in the former).

To return to the principle of the multi-axial classification:

		How has it been?	How is it now?
1	Mental life: ideas, attitudes thinking, feeling and behaviour		
2	Developmental ability or disorder		
3	Intellectual ability or retardation		
4	Physical health and ability		
5	Family, social and cultural life, expectations, opportunities and pressures		

The current environment continued: the referral process. Of all these factors, one aspect of the environment tends to receive less attention than it should, and that is the *process of referral*, i.e. the process by which a boy or girl, with whatever problems or lack of them, is selected as possibly having a psychiatric disorder.

Even in circles that accept the social contribution to disorder, there is a tendency to exempt from consideration the motivation of the professional making the preliminary diagnosis: 'this child may be mentally disturbed'. It is as though parents, uncles, aunts, cousins, siblings, teachers and others all make their contribution to what has gone wrong, but once someone says 'this child has a problem' it is as if a bell has been rung, a truce called, and everyone goes to their corner (except the child!) while the psychiatrist is called in to diagnose the boy or girl.

Bruggen[13, 14] has described an approach to adolescents referred for admission to his unit which attempts to deal with the total referral process. The title of one of the papers in which he describes his style of work explains itself: 'The reason for admission as a focus of work'. He and his colleagues do not believe in making a clinical diagnosis and using psychiatric authority to recommend the child's admission. Rather whatever may or may not be 'wrong' with the child, Bruggen's team focuses on why the family (or social worker or 'outside' psychiatric team) cannot cope, and offer group support (with admission of the child if necessary) until they can. It is a difficult way to work and causes much misunderstanding and complaint but illustrates this aspect of diagnosis nicely.

It is of course true that in recent years there has been a tendency to focus on the 'sick family' rather than the child, but the result is often similar, with the family, instead of the child, being referred on for ever more expert assessment and treatment. In the formality of referral there is a tendency to leave out such questions as: what difficulties has the *professional making the referral* run into? might it be more helpful all round to help him (or her) carry on, rather than book the child and family in for an 'assessment', which may well be the third, or fourth?

The multi-axial diagnostic system already described, may of course include the diagnosis that under the heading 'clinical psychiatric syndrome' nothing is individually wrong with the child (although psychiatrists unfortunately tend to be reluctant to use this 'zero' category). The diagnosis may well be:

Axis One	– Clinical psychiatric syndrome	No abnormality
Axis Two	– Developmental state	,,
Axis Three	– Intellectual level	,,
Axis Four	– Physical state	,,
Axis Five	– Family discord and major problems at school	*Problems*

But in drawing these conclusions, we tend not to include in the diagnostic assessment: but with what should the parents be able to cope? And if they can't, *with what degree of family disturbance should the social worker (or other professional) be able to cope?* Similarly, what is the 'normal' degree of disturbance with which a teacher should cope? Or with what degree of anxiety and uncertainty among teaching staff should a headmaster, or school counsellor, or educational psychologist, be able to cope?

What is psychiatric disorder?

It is the successive 'breakdown' of a sequence of normal social coping mechanisms, and then the breakdown of a sequence of increasingly specialised coping resources, that lead the child inexorably towards a source of help which traditionally is supposed to combine a magical cure or special understanding with a willingness to put up with anything: psychiatry. One definition of psychiatric disorder might be 'that extreme or deviant thinking, feeling and behaviour with which ordinary individual and community coping mechanisms, including special efforts at care, education and control, cannot cope'.

Edmund Leach has put it another way:[56] the community deals with its most challenging innovators in three ways – by putting them in prisons, in mental hospitals or in universities. If one includes in the last category established academic and creative people generally, I think this is true.

If a group of strangely dressed young people were found doing bizarre, extrovert and perhaps distasteful things in the local high street one Saturday afternoon, the chances are that the vast majority of passers-by would explain the situation in one of three ways: (i) that the group were 'bad' (shouldn't be allowed) – the police should be called; (ii) that they were 'mad' ('ought to be put away'); (iii) that perhaps they were a bunch of actors or artists from the local college.

If a teacher has a child in his class who is behaving in a way quite out of the ordinary, yet not apparently creatively, he will naturally use his own experience and skills to understand the child and try to guide the child's odd behaviour into a more socially acceptable and appropriate pattern. If he can't, after trying for some time, he may call in more help. An educational psychologist, for example, may think: this child *is* behaving oddly, and on balance more than is manageable in this class. Perhaps he should be in another class, another school, or referred to the local psychiatric clinic. Before making this decision, he may well have tried methods in the classroom with the teacher's collaboration, to deal with the child's behaviour and not succeeded.

The point being made is *not* that a line should not be drawn, beyond which certain behaviour is regarded as eccentric, disruptive or unmanageable. Of course it must. But *where* it is drawn – the point at which the decision is made that the problem is a psychiatric one – depends on the capacity and understanding and resources of the professional on the spot, *and this varies*.

If, in my psychiatric unit, I decide that my colleagues (and therefore I) cannot cope any longer with a child who is, say, repeatedly setting light to his bed, this says something about myself and my colleagues as well as about the child. Could the child really be contained better elsewhere? Is there anything else we might be able to do if we thought more about the problem? Are we anxious because we really think we cannot cope, or is it because the very small chance of disaster is one that our institution and the community is not prepared to accept, and therefore if the unit is burned down and people hurt or even killed we will not be supported by those to whom we are responsible?

This aspect of the diagnosis of a problem applies to a large number of difficult situations with children. For example a teacher is not confident his headmaster will back him up if he presses on, trying to help a promiscuous girl and she accuses him of assault. Perhaps he thinks the headmaster would have trusted him but be unable to defend him against the PTA, the school governors, or even the Press. A social worker feels she could manage a mother threatening assault on her child, and a trusting relationship is building up (which is why the woman has been able to express her aggressive fears), but her seniors have laid down a 'procedure' for child abuse which must be followed, and includes removing from the social worker the professional right to take a carefully and responsibly calculated risk.

But, at another extreme, a teacher, or a social worker, or a house-parent may be adequately backed up by their colleagues, but over-anxious about the case because of their own background, personality, experience and skills.

All this is not to 'blame' the adult who refers a child for help. Quite the reverse: it takes competence and maturity to know how and when to ask for help. But in diagnosing the child and the family, some understanding must also be reached about what the other adults involved have not been able to do, and what they could be able to do with the right information, advice and support.

Consultation is the technical term for the process by which one professional helps another in their work. As the total situation is diagnosed, and we begin to think about what sorts of management we have up our professional sleeves for the child (treatment, training, care or control) we should also think whether consultation might help the referring professional cope with the case, or an aspect of the case. This will be taken up again in chapter 7.

Medical versus social models of disorder

The idea of psychiatric disorder representing social as well as clinical phenomena is not new; for example, see the writings of Foucault, Lewis, Rosen, Laing and others.[32],[55],[58],[77]

Beware of simplistic arguments in either direction, because the issue is a very complicated one. To say all these problems are social is as potentially tyrannical as to hold that they are all medical, and both attitudes are equally unhelpful. There are occasions when there *is* something 'wrong' with the individual boy or girl, and the community has a right to expect the professional (psychiatrist or other worker) to establish what this is, and what can be done to help. As mentioned earlier, this is the essence of the medical model. Equally, there are occasions when psychiatric disorder has been attributed to the child when the real and perhaps reversible problems lie elsewhere. Again, something can be done about this too, but perhaps by family or social work, perhaps by major changes in the school or home, perhaps by wider social education and reform. The psychiatrist can help establish these other needs and resources by the important function of saying what is *not* a psychiatric problem. The psychiatrist's task is first to clarify problems in a whole range of dimensions and then to say which, if any, he can do something about, as a doctor.

Diagnosis in practice

Different psychiatric teams work very differently. The archetypal approach is something like this: a psychiatrist sees the child, a psychologist then sees him too, for intellectual assessment, and a social worker sees the parents. What the psychiatrist does when he sees the child depends on the child's age and problems and capacity to discuss things. Sufficient to say that the psychiatrist has to take time to get to know the boy or girl, through conversation and perhaps play with toys, drawing and other methods. A 'one-off' diagnosis on the basis of a series of clinical questions is not enough. Problems can take time to clarify; but with experience child psychiatrists can often conclude fairly quickly if a boy's or girl's responses, mood and thinking seem to be basically normal. The three workers then put together psychiatric state, intellectual level and family history and circumstances.

This system has not stood the test of time too well. Many psychologists have a far wider range of skills than simply 'testing', and recent developments in understanding the importance of family dynamics have made it useful to see the whole family operating together, at least for some of the time given to the assessment.

Who attends?

Some psychiatric teams will only see the whole family all together; others never do. On the one hand, the family approach is among the most important recent developments in child psychiatry and a valuable tool for both diagnosis and treatment. On the other, it has also become fashionable, which means that people will try it because it is radical, new, different, vaguely 'open' and democratic, and therefore good. But for some families and some problems a child and parents are more helpfully assessed separately. Some enthusiastic monotherapists energetically insist that their style is the right one, and may refuse to adapt their approach to what the child and family want, claiming that what they *want* is not what they *need*. There is something in this, but there is also more than a touch of time-honoured professional arrogance too.

What *is* to be deprecated is the sloppy system by which, in recent times, fathers were rarely or never seen in child guidance clinics because they were busy at work, and only the mother was considered free to come along. If the father cannot get away from work to help sort out his child's problem, at least initially, he may need help to do so: e.g. to be reminded that he is a most important person in the family's life. He may welcome a note for his employer explaining that he is needed on this occasion. He should not be browbeaten into turning up. The point is that the child psychiatric team should not too readily fall into the trap – admittedly a rapidly dating one – of going along with the assumption that a child's problem is not a serious matter for the father.

Children tend to know more or less what is going on in a family, and have anxieties of their own, strongly coloured and usually made worse by fears and fantasies. So it is helpful in most cases if the referred child's brothers and sisters are seen too, at that first interview, to contribute to our understanding of how the whole family operates, and to be given a simple explanation in plain English about what is going on, and what is to be done. Often, this also reveals when undue pressure is being put on another child in the family and also which children are special sources of comfort and strength.

The system we use in my own unit is basically as follows, it is deliberately adaptable, and includes as a focus the process of referral.

(a) First, all new referrals are discussed by the clinical team – psychiatrists, psychologists, social workers, nurses and teachers. This is a teaching and learning occasion as well as a decision-making meeting; if urgent decisions are needed about particular cases these will already have been made.

(b) *Either* one of the team arranges to discuss the case further with the referring professional *or* the child and family are given an appointment. Meanwhile we seek permission from the family to get school reports, etc.

(c) When the child and family arrive, they are seen together by the people taking part in that morning's assessment – doctor, social worker, sometimes psychologist, and one of the nurses if admission is a strong possibility, to clarify briefly why they have come. Sometimes this is the first time that this is made clear to the child and even, sometimes, to the family.

(d) The doctor and social worker see the family together for part of the time and later, depending on the problem and how the interview is progressing, the social worker continues separately with the parents and the doctor with the child. The parents may have indicated they would prefer a discussion with the social worker away from the child; this need for the grown-ups to talk privately will be explained to the child. Alternatively, the doctor may feel the child has a problem or abnormality better assessed separately. This stage might include the child having formal psychological testing, or a physical examination. Electro-encephalographic (E.E.G.)[39] and other tests of physical health may be decided upon too.

(e) The clinical team and any 'outside' professionals who are attending meet to discuss how best to proceed.

(f) This is then discussed with the whole family, plans made and appointments fixed.

Conclusions

All this may seem cumbersome, and is certainly a long way removed from the traditional medical referral by which a family doctor books a patient into a clinic and sends a covering letter beginning 'Thank you for seeing . . .'. But it is right that this be so because, as explained earlier, the indications for psychiatric assessment and treatment are arbitrary in the extreme, many children have psychiatric disorder unnecessarily attributed to them, and many who are referred do not in fact need to be seen. This statement may be misunderstood and needs qualification. I am not suggesting that a psychiatric clinic should be remote and unhelpful, but quite the reverse. The members of a specialist psychiatric team should make themselves more accessible, not less, to people – parents or professionals – wanting advice, but the process of formally booking a child into a clinic for a detailed diagnostic assessment should be a later step, not the initial one. This applies even more strongly to children and adolescents referred for admission to hospital. A rapid and helpful response to the adult concerned about the child is needed, but the idea that the child needs to be got rapidly 'into treatment' almost always is a misunderstanding about treatment and about the child.

There are of course exceptions, in particular the very few children acutely ill and in danger with an acute psychotic illness or suicidal depression. Moreover, the theoretical standpoint proposed does not prevent an individual member of the psychiatric team from taking an on-the-spot decision in an emergency; rather, it enhances the quality of the sort of preliminary diagnosis he is able to make, e.g. on the basis of an urgent telephone call.

Child and adolescent psychiatric clinics are often accused of having too long a waiting list. But for the minority of children and families who *really* need a thorough assessment of what has gone wrong over five, ten or fifteen years, some two hours or more may have to be spent in listening carefully to what has gone on, and finding out what the child and his family are like. One of the special resources a psychiatrist must be able to give his patients is *time*. He and the patient need this as much as the surgeon and his patient need a sterile space to work in. A child psychiatric service should make time for those who need it by dealing competently (not dismissively) with the majority who do not.

Child and adolescent in-patient units, in particular, are often accused of being selective. So they should be. But only if they are as generous and responsive in offering information, advice, consultation and support as they are parsimonious in picking out the relatively small number of boys and girls who really need a psychiatrist.[99, 100]

5

Child Psychiatry II:
Treatment

What do child psychiatrists do?

Having stressed the case for carefully selecting children
for psychiatry, we should consider what psychiatry has
to offer. Later chapters take up again the theme of
the proper role of child and adolescent psychiatry. This
chapter outlines the treatments and methods of management potentially available to the child and adolescent
psychiatric team, without at this stage discussing which
members of the clinical team should do what.

The point about methods of treatment being *potentially*
available is an important one. What the local child
psychiatric clinic actually provides depends partly on the
personal preferences of the people who work there, and
in particular its leadership (of which more later), and
partly on what the Health, Social Service and Education
departments have been willing and able to provide in the
way of resources. One team will favour family therapy
and perhaps offer little else. Another may be reluctant to
prescribe drugs. Another will tend to see the referred
child for individual psychotherapy while the team's
social worker sees the child's mother. Most clinics do
not have direct access to in-patient places; and when
there is an in-patient unit for children or adolescents
nearby the relationship between the two clinical teams
is not always an easy one because of disagreements

about criteria for admission to hospital, among other things.[99, 100]

The distinction between diagnosis and treatment implied by the headings of chapters 4 and 5 can be misleading. Of course a diagnostic formulation has to be made, a hypothesis about what has happened to the boy or girl and what response might be helpful, but it is unusual for the simple formula 'this is the disorder and this is its treatment' to be adequate. Each individual is unique, and in each case, inevitably, treatment is something of an experiment. A 'one-off' diagnosis is a provisional hypothesis about the child and his or her situation, and the effects of treatment have to be monitored along the five axes already described. Psychotherapy every week may begin to help a child with a particular intrapsychic difficulty but his social functioning may continue to be a problem. Drugs may dramatically improve a state of high anxiety but impair ability to learn at school. Treatment, therefore, requires continuing assessment, which means continuing diagnosis. This is the medical meaning of the term management: monitoring the effects of the various ways in which one tries to help.

Categories of treatment

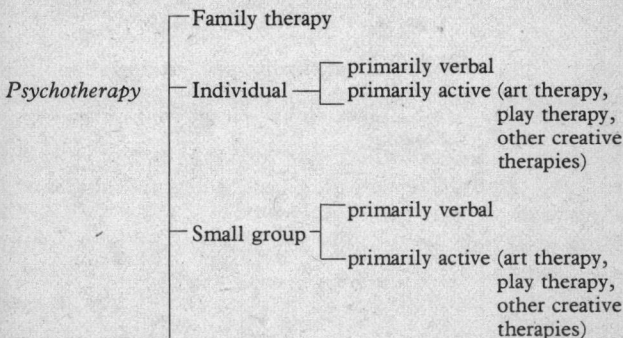

Psychotherapy

- Family therapy
- Individual
  - primarily verbal
  - primarily active (art therapy, play therapy, other creative therapies)
- Small group
  - primarily verbal
  - primarily active (art therapy, play therapy, other creative therapies)

Categories of treatment – *continued*

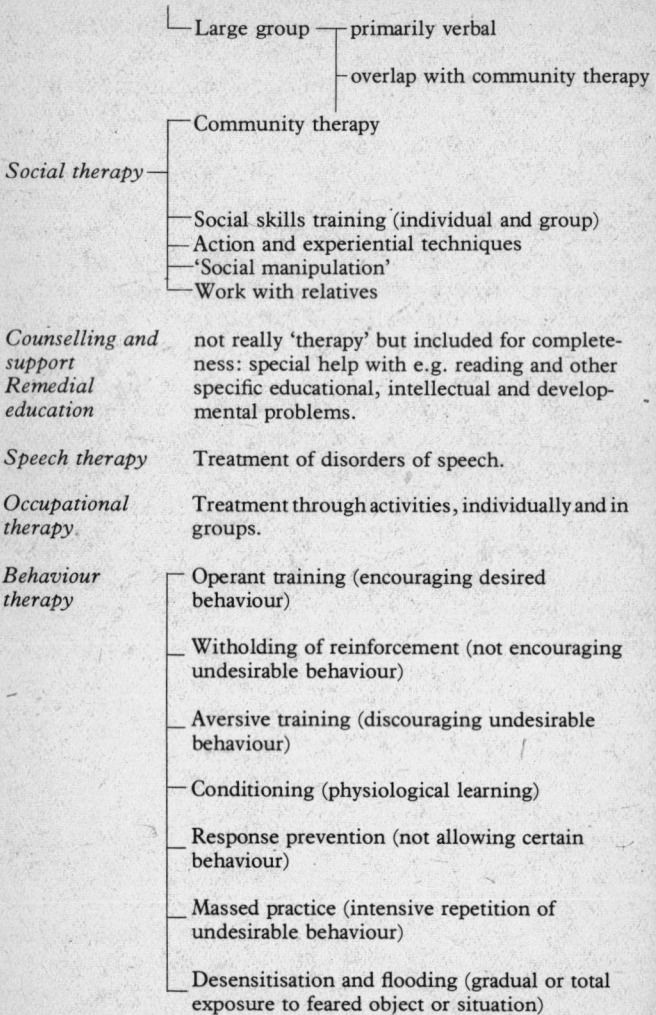

        └─ Large group ─┬─ primarily verbal

                         └─ overlap with community therapy

        ┌─ Community therapy

Social therapy ─┤

        ├─ Social skills training (individual and group)
        ├─ Action and experiential techniques
        ├─ 'Social manipulation'
        └─ Work with relatives

Counselling and support
Remedial education — not really 'therapy' but included for completeness: special help with e.g. reading and other specific educational, intellectual and developmental problems.

Speech therapy — Treatment of disorders of speech.

Occupational therapy — Treatment through activities, individually and in groups.

Behaviour therapy
    ┌─ Operant training (encouraging desired behaviour)

    ├─ Witholding of reinforcement (not encouraging undesirable behaviour)

    ├─ Aversive training (discouraging undesirable behaviour)

    ├─ Conditioning (physiological learning)

    ├─ Response prevention (not allowing certain behaviour)

    ├─ Massed practice (intensive repetition of undesirable behaviour)

    └─ Desensitisation and flooding (gradual or total exposure to feared object or situation)

Categories of treatment – *continued*

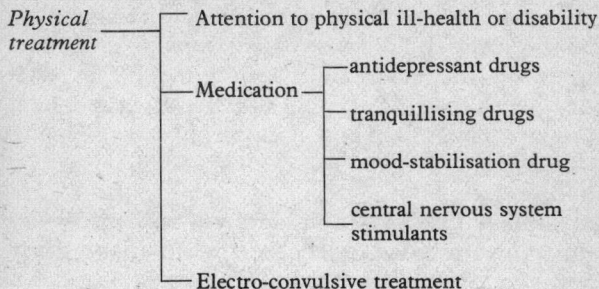

Physical treatment
- Attention to physical ill-health or disability
- Medication
  - antidepressant drugs
  - tranquillising drugs
  - mood-stabilisation drug
  - central nervous system stimulants
- Electro-convulsive treatment

Nursing See below.

Where treated?
In the home and/or at school.
Attending an out-patient clinic.
Attending a day centre or specialised schooling.
Away from home in a hospital or other therapeutic setting, or in a residential school.

Treated by whom?
By the child and adolescent psychiatrist or one of his or her immediate colleagues in the clinical team.
By a non-clinical professional, e.g. residential child care worker, or teacher.
By the parents, or by the family.

This is not a totally neat and tidy classification. Thus treatment away from home implies the need for treatment primarily by people other than parents and teachers, for example. The idea of treatment by parents or teachers may not be a familiar one; it is an important part of child psychiatric practice[3,4,50,91] and brings into the consideration of how a psychiatric team can operate various collaborative approaches. This is the subject of chapter 7.

Treatment approaches outlined

A detailed account of these approaches to treatment is beyond the scope and purpose of this book. What follow are notes on the basic aims and principles of each category, with particular reference to aspects which cause misunderstanding and controversy.

Psychotherapy

Many people will tell you confidently what is necessary to train in and practise psychotherapy; there are many different versions, and a good deal of controversy, including the doubt frequently expressed about whether this form of treatment works at all. On the one hand practitioners can be found who exaggerate the advantages of psychotherapy in general and their own favourite brand (the one they have trained in at considerable cost) in particular. On the other, there are people who dismiss psychotherapy out of hand as if it could not work; some academic psychiatrists and psychologists take this approach, and they appear to hold the view that it is not possible, or likely, for someone to influence profoundly another by his contact and affect the way his ideas, attitudes and personality develop; an odd notion for teachers to adhere to.

Basic to psychotherapy, in my view, is the relationship that develops between therapist and patient, and the essence of this relationship (if it is going to be helpful) is that it is both *challenging* and *safe*. It is safe in the sense that the patient – in this case the child or adolescent – believes correctly that he is going to be properly looked after and not suddenly abandoned or made the recipient of neurotic reactions by the therapist – inappropriate anger or anxiety for example, perhaps leading to the abandonment of treatment, or for example, the clumsy handling of a difficult topic. Often this sense of the therapist providing a 'safe base' is reinforced by punctiliousness about the place, time and timing of the sessions: they are reliable and predictable.

It is challenging in that the psychotherapist, especially with young people, tends not to take the caricatured role of the psychotherapist: passive, non-committal, largely silent, perhaps asleep. Most child and adolescent psychotherapy is active, conversational and lively, with humour and disagreement and revelation of the psychotherapist's feelings and attitudes allowed. A psychotherapist may not be practising psychotherapy if he tells a delinquent patient that he is a little villain, or words to that effect, but he may be right to tell him angrily that he, personally, finds his behaviour infuriating or whatever. There is a difference. Psychotherapists hope and believe that their training (which often includes a personal analysis) enables their reactions to their patients to be unfettered by past hang-ups, so that their responses are a nice balance between healthy spontaneity and useful intervention. Thus with a difficult child they will allow themselves to express anger, if that is how the child makes them feel, and if responding angrily will help; but they will hope to be able to avoid the unhelpful punitiveness of one sort of parental response, and the over-indulgence and permissiveness of another. Wyss[118] concludes his excellent review of schools of dynamic psychology with the observation that psychotherapy boils down to perception and love; but it take *both*, and often what passes for psychotherapy is overloaded one way or the other.

How does this differ from common sense and good parenting? Common sense, by definition, is that which is commonly believed and practised, and includes all the usual woolly human inconsistencies and muddle which the majority of children take in their stride. A boy or girl may be walloped for misbehaviour one day, and laughed at for the same behaviour the next. Parents often give children mixed messages – the famous 'double-bind' – and it doesn't cause schizophrenia, although the notion induced guilt and paranoia in a generation of informed, middle-class parents. Most children are resilient, and cope with less than perfect handling. But some do not, and the task of the psychotherapist, if psychotherapy is prescribed, is to set up a series of regular and probably frequent sessions in which close attention is paid to that child's developing relationship with the therapist and what sort of moods and ideas and behaviour emerges as the relationship develops, and what it all means. The problems which arise (e.g. a child's sadness and sensitiveness, for which he was referred) emerge as hopelessness *about the sessions* and suspiciousness and vulnerability *towards the therapist*, and the latter tries to deal with these real, not recalled, feelings when they meet.

Part of the discipline of properly conducted psychotherapy is careful reflection about the content of the sessions. More experienced psychotherapists 'consult with themselves', others attend supervision sessions. The advice and accurate predictions (about the sessions) from a good supervisor can be genuinely impressive. What remains controversial is the extent to which things learned and attributes acquired by the child in psychotherapy generalise to ordinary life. The aim is that psychotherapy helps the child grow into a different sort of young person by being able to be a different sort of person in the psychotherapeutic relationship. How often this is achieved is an open question, and when it is achieved it is not *proved* that the massive investment of psychotherapy and psychotherapeutic training was essential. Perhaps the jargon and the training simply helps the therapist persist long enough with a child it is hard to understand or like.

Some psychotherapy with older and more articulate children and adolescents is largely verbal, if more conversational in style than orthodox psychotherapy as often practised with adults. But for many children and adolescents, and certainly young children, creative activity, games and play as the media for expressing and coping with feelings, is more important. Hence child psychiatrists accumulate in their rooms paper, pens, paints, dolls' houses, toys and so on, and if they are lucky and well endowed a sand-pit to play in too. It is easy to make light of such media. In fact a child who could never articulate, and perhaps hardly conceive, that she fears her parents have no time for her, might reveal her feelings by populating the clinic's dolls' house with all the little figures but leaving out the adult dolls; using the dolls and dolls' house the therapist and child together can make up stories about what's going on, how it feels, and how to cope with it.

These techniques are not merely diagnostic manoeuvres. A common misconception about the use of art in psychotherapy, for example, is that the psychotherapist knowingly points out the patient's hitherto unrevealed 'complexes' as shown by the way he or she has drawn a dog or a tree. Sometimes there is a smattering of truth about an observation of this sort, but it is not the whole truth, and what is more revealing is, again, the relationship between patient, therapist and, in this case, the piece of creative work being attempted.

A depressed little girl is invited to join in with her therapist in playing with clay. She smiles and declines, preferring to watch. The therapist lets her watch while he plays about with the clay himself, clearly having fun, and after a while tosses the girl a bit of clay and asks her to 'make the tail' while he makes the rest of some small animal. She very hesitatingly makes an elongated scrap of clay; the therapist bangs it onto the back of the clay monkey, sits back, gazes at it quizzically and pronounces it no use to man or beast, drawing the little girl into the joke. He pretends to tear his hair and gives her another bit of clay, and they start again.

This is not supposed to be a solemn illustration of a leap forward in the psychotherapy of a child's depression;

it may represent only a drop in the ocean of work done. For whatever reason, the little girl has been taught to hide her feelings, especially angry and sad ones, and is fearful of making mistakes. If she can find in the therapist someone with whom she can relax and be playful, and risk and indeed make mistakes, over time she may be able to be a different sort of person, at least with him. But note that although the therapist is kind and accepting to the girl, he doesn't accept all she does, even in the small business of the badly made tail. It would be bogus to enthuse over 'what a lovely tail' if the little girl knows it isn't, and couldn't be since she didn't enjoy making it and wanted only to get the bit of clay off her hands at the earliest moment.

The use of art as a medium for psychotherapy is a large and still developing subject, and this is only a glimpse of it.

All this makes psychotherapy seem rather calculating, and up to a point it is, though in theory, and sometimes in practice, psychotherapeutic training may help an individual react in a warm, reasonable, encouraging and genuine way, as did the therapist in this example. The 'common sense' response to the little girl of saying 'oh, what a lovely little tail you've made' when it wasn't, is *not* encouraging, and more likely to be indicative of the clumsy and casual way adults quite often treat children, and which, fortunately, doesn't matter too much to most. Psychotherapy training no doubt helps some professionals to be more helpfully 'natural', while others respond helpfully to their patients by a constant process of thinking through what is going on. Either way, psychotherapists, especially those in training, need time to reflect carefully about their sessions with their patients, alone or, preferably, with others.

How does this differ from 'ordinary' good relationships and skilled handling? Mainly in the degree of formality and the extra degrees of technical understanding needed when a child has been unable to learn and

develop emotionally from normal handling. The psychotherapist usually specifies set sessions at set times, and
spends time and effort in thinking about what happens
in those sessions, with a supervisor if he is relatively
inexperienced. The degree to which 'interpretations' are
used – i.e. translating what the patient says or does into
a symbolic language that makes sense to the psychotherapist, and enables him to make sense of the patient's
speech and behaviour – varies with the psychotherapist.
Some people, including the author, believe that such
interpretations are for the therapist's use, not the
patient's, and help the therapist understand what is
going on in the relationship. He doesn't 'interpret' to
the child what he thinks the child means, but rather
adapts his own behaviour. Thus he would not say
'you're inhibited because you are fearful of parental
authority figures', but will *behave* as if this is true for
this child, just as the therapist in the above example *did*
assert his own adult authority about the puny tail, but in
a friendly, non-punitive, honest way.

Individual psychotherapy is an attempt to deal with
the child's supposed internal, individual emotional and
personality difficulties as revealed by what he or she says
and does and by the relationship with the therapist. The
child in the example lacks confidence and is unhappy,
and it is assumed that this problem is, as it were, 'carried
around' within her, to be revealed when any relationship scratches the surface.

But its origin may well be in the way she has been
talked to and handled by her parents, and if the girl were
to be seen with her whole family *the process by which she
is undermined and made miserable, and sustained in this
condition, may be seen in action.*

It may be seen in her smiling, resigned look when her
overwrought mother tells the therapist that her husband
won't come to the clinic – 'he's not interested; he's very
busy at work at the moment'. If and when he is persuaded
to attend it may be clear that he prefers the company of

his two brisk, matter-of-fact sons to his miserable wife and daughter. In *family therapy* the therapist tries to deal not with the individual child's psychodynamics, but with the processes in the family that maintain its members in positions and attitudes that, one way or another, are causing emotional pain and disability. As with individual psychotherapy, there is an assumption that serious work is being done, and that sessions take place punctually and regularly, with the right people there. (How many of child psychiatry's failures result from half-heartedness on the part of some of its practitioners, subscribing to the superficially modest but really rather arrogant maxim 'it doesn't really matter what you do'?)

Group psychotherapy may be undertaken with a number of children who happen to be together anyway, e.g. in a class or home, or who are selected to take part in a particular series of sessions. Again, the principle is that individual assets and difficulties will emerge from the group in due course (as in the familiar theme of many novels) and the group therapist uses the group, by his interventions, to establish trust, enable social experiments, 'games' and relationships to develop, and try to influence them. The aggressive child may be made, firmly, to sit still and be quiet; the inhibited child helped to speak up for himself; the touchy, sensitive child who assumes his own unpopularity may be shown how he makes it difficult for other people to be friendly with him. A group for children or adolescents is more productive when activity-based rather than purely verbal; not that children's groups remain seated and talking for long in any case.[101]

Psychodynamic theory, the psychotherapeutic treatments that have developed from it, and their adaptation to the needs of disturbed children is a very large subject indeed. It should be read around, reliance on one theorist's or practitioner's particular approach being misleading. Some of the references given in the list of references (p. 193) will be found useful guides to the way psychodynamicists think and work, and to further reading.

Social therapy

By its use of social expectations and pressures, small and large group psychotherapy with children and adolescents overlaps with the use of the *community*, and usually residential community, as a therapeutic setting. There is a good deal of misunderstanding about what constitutes a *therapeutic community*. Occasionally adults form truly democratic self-help groups without professional help and hierarchies, but usually the hierarchy is there but lies low. Children and adolescents should not be expected to take full responsibility for themselves, though older, better adjusted children must of course be helped to share in taking responsibility; most psychiatric settings for children and adolescents which have some claim to be therapeutic environments mean by this that the staff operate the home so that its various rules and expectations and sources of love, care and discipline have treatment goals. This means that it is not simply casually well-meaning, but like psychotherapy operates according to a principle, and its day-to-day operation is discussed and thought through.

It is difficult to say where psychotherapy ends and social therapy begins. One could argue that any psychotherapy which uses the relationship between people (i.e. as is usually the case) is really a social therapy. In practice the term is usually applied where the social group that has other functions too (e.g. as a place to live, or learn academically) *also* operates as a setting for individual therapy, using relationships, responsibilities and expectations of the community as the medium for the emergence of problems and their solution.

Social skills training is a valuable technique applicable to adolescents. Specific difficulties are agreed upon –

e.g. lack of assertiveness, or lack of confidence in interviews – and in a small group, or with the therapist alone, the patient practises doing what he cannot usually do.

This is as good a point as any to mention 'action' techniques that may be used in psychotherapy and social therapy, and indeed in training. In *role play*, the people involved act the parts relevant to the issue; it can be a sobering experience for a misbehaving adolescent to be cajoled into playing the part of a teacher trying to control an unruly class consisting of his peers and some clinic staff. Role play is concerned more with overt behaviour and relationships; a related technique, *psycho-drama*, is a more emotive and sensitive approach in which, with due precautions, the individual is helped by other people to act out and experience feelings and fantasies, perhaps in relationship to his or her family. In *sculpting*, posture, position and expression of the group is used to express what may not be expressed well in words. A family which claims to be 'very close' may turn out, when a member is helped by the therapist to 'place', say, parents and siblings, to be all looking in different directions and yards apart.

These techniques are gaining popularity. In skilled hands they can be remarkable aids to psychotherapy and social therapy, and for training in both. They are also highly attractive to the histrionic and superficial and can result in misleading conclusions and indeed a good deal of pain when used with enthusiasm but without wisdom and responsibility.

Social manipulation is a terrible term, but more or less accurately describes the selection of a particular environment, or its modification, in order to help a child. It is included for completeness, but of course is the antithesis of treatment; the situation is being changed, not the child, either in the hope that in the new setting the boy or girl will be better able to develop emotionally and in other ways, or because only against the background of a new setting will one or other treatment stand a chance of helping.

Thus a child may be recommended for a place in a children's home, perhaps supported by being taken into care under the provisions of the Children's and Young Person's Act. Sometimes parents are unable or unwilling to assert helpful parental authority, or neglect a child in some other way – reception into care, and the guidance and advice of a social worker, can be useful without the child actually leaving home; in such cases the authority of the law, and the implications of community concern implied, help child and parents. A child may be recommended for boarding education – not necessarily of a specialised sort. To return to the model introduced on p. 28, it is at this point that concepts of treatment meet concepts of special care.

Work with relatives
Therapeutic work with the child's parents, or occasionally with one or more brothers or sisters, should be distinguished from family therapy. In family therapy the whole group living together are seen. Sometimes separate work needs to be done with one or other parent, or both together. This may be psychotherapeutic work, perhaps marital or sexual therapy, or psychiatric treatment for parental illness, which is closely associated with emotional and conduct problems in children.[79, 81] Also important is helping parents manage disturbed children more competently, as with autistic children.[91]

Counselling and support

'*Supportive psychotherapy*' is a commonly used term. Some practitioners of psychotherapy favour primarily supportive psychotherapy. I feel that psychotherapy should be regarded as a special treatment technique with its own jargon, rules and goals, for good or ill, and that 'support' is a kind enough and sensible thing for a professional to offer a child or family without regrading it as 'therapy'.

Counselling should be distinguished from psycho-therapy, and Newsome[67, 68] has attempted this admirably. The young person, usually an adolescent, is not 'diagnosed' or 'treated' but as much initiative as possible is left with the person concerned about the initiation of sessions, the issue on which he wants help and clarification, he is helped to explore matters for himself, and decides when to stop.

Remedial education

Here treatment meets education, and of course they overlap, but as argued elsewhere the fundamental differences between their core functions should be recognised and clarified. Remedial education may help a child learn whose educational attainment has fallen behind; the skill of the teacher is in working with both emotional and intellectual impediments to learning. But the reverse can also operate, when a child's emotional problems are helped by experiencing, perhaps for the first time, the stimulus, rewards and sense of achievement of developing academic and creative skills.

Conduct disorders, relationship problems (with peers and adults) and educational difficulty, with or without specific learning problems, frequently co-exist. All children need education, but some children's needs are more special than others; whenever the problems and possible help for a disturbed child are considered, it is always important to consider what difficulties (social as well as academic) are revealed in the classroom and playground, and what solutions may be found there.

Speech therapy

We tend to take the comprehension and production of language for granted; it is an absolutely remarkable capacity and skill, and abnormalities in its development are inseparably bound up with the functioning of the nervous system and with mental life. Speech therapy is perhaps best known as a treatment prescribed for relatively simple disorders in the articulation of speech, but understanding the nature of language and speech problems and what to do for them is an important and expanding field.[44, 82, 119]

Occupational therapy

For historical reasons occupational therapy is a prominent treatment method in hospital settings (both for in-patients and day-patients) but features little in child psychiatric or child 'guidance' clinics. As with other professions there is an overlap with what other people do, and the skills of many occupational therapists have much in common with those of specialist teachers, play therapists, creative therapists and social therapists. The essence of the specialty is two-edged: on the one hand, using such occupations as cooking, typing, craft work, gardening, looking after animals and simply playing, as the medium through which children and adolescents learn to acquire skills, confidence, stimulation and the capacity to organise themselves and co-operate with others; and on the other hand, helping a young person who is being treated by other methods to rehearse and practise the process of deciding on leisure activities and a career, and going about instituting them. Occupational therapy is about how to work and play, and many emotionally disabled young people enter adult life able to do neither competently.

Behaviour therapy

Like psychotherapy, behaviour therapy (or behavioural psychotherapy, as some practitioners prefer to call it) is a very large subject, and to understand what it can offer, and its limitations too, requires reasonably wide reading of its theory and practice.[65, 120] The treatment techniques themselves, however, can be commendably straightforward and applied by people with relatively limited training. The other side of this particular coin, however, is that while the target symptoms may be competently treated, related matters to do with school, the family and how the child feels also need attention, and this requires a different sort of skill.

In essence, behaviour therapy is not concerned with ideas, feelings and motives but with behaviour, i.e. overt, observable symptoms and behaviour patterns. This is why it irritates many psychodynamic therapists, who believe that the root cause of such behaviour lies in the unconscious psyche, and if the child isn't helped at this level, suppressing or changing behaviour will simply result in the same problem reappearing in a different form: stop a child bed wetting by behavioural means, and he will become conduct-disordered instead.

Undoubtedly family and individual problems are expressed in different ways from time to time, and indeed any treatment may not work, and the child get worse in one or other way; but there is no evidence for the supposition that as one symptom is suppressed by behavioural means, another takes its place. As shown in chapter 3, life isn't that simple. A child, ashamed and miserable about his bed wetting, may be able to achieve a new emotional and social equilibrium once it is brought to a halt by what psychodynamic purists would regard as superficial means.

The whole argument is a spurious one, only having validity if the contending sides really believe on the one hand that the human individual does not have the capacity to develop behavioural habits which are self-perpetuating, whatever the psyche does; or on the other that his or her behaviour is never affected significantly by largely unconscious and non-rational motives and feelings. Both can be true of all people, and correspondingly the patterns we label as disorders can be based on one or the other or a little of both.

In *operant training* desired behaviour is encouraged; rewards are more effective than punishment, and to give a child his pocket money (or a proportion of it) because of a reasonably well behaved week is likely to be more effective than stopping it for naughty behaviour, at least for the emotionally disturbed. Behavioural principles can reveal the flaws in 'common sense'. A parent or teacher may get furious with a naughty child and even thump him, leaving him alone when he is well behaved. But this sort of child may be particularly inept at getting along by himself, and his background may make him more fearful of being neglected than of being hit. He may respond far better to being given lots of attention when 'good', and being ignored as far as this is possible when 'bad'. This approach, in which scraps of 'positive' behaviour are noted, focused upon, encouraged, and, to use the jargon, 'shaped up', can be most effective. It is painstaking, persistent work. With some children this approach taken by a teacher, perhaps with a psychologist's advice, can have a dramatically improving effect. At the other extreme, a very disturbed child may need to be in a residential unit where this sort of line can be taken systematically around the clock. Similarly rewards conditional upon weight-gain are used for young people with anorexia nervosa.

Witholding of reinforcement is complementary to this, and a well-known example is 'time out', a procedure where a child who is, say, having a tantrum or behaving aggressively is immediately removed from the scene (which is assumed to have factors within it provoking and encouraging this behaviour) and put in *and kept in* a 'time out' room for a few minutes. He isn't kept there for longer, but goes straight back there the next time he behaves that way; and so on. Again, it can be effective, and even welcomed by the child, as a controlling but non-retributory procedure that supervenes when he becomes chaotic with rage and fear.

Aversive training, or punishment, is even more unfashionable. The most striking example I have heard of is the use of painful though non-damaging electric

shocks for a mentally-retarded child who was systematically blinding and killing himself by persistently beat-
ing his head against a wall.

Of all forms of behaviour therapy, the latter two
approaches – in particular time out and punishment –
cause the most controversy. They can be and are abused,
and 'time out' can be allowed to blur with locking-up
('seclusion' is the term), which is control rather than
treatment. Nevertheless it may be the only way to make
the child manageable and, more important, the only way
to contain the child in a setting which keeps him out of
worse trouble and offers other forms of treatment too.
People who object strenuously to such approaches often
have no alternatives to offer themselves. (The story is
told that R D Laing, taking a discussion after showing a
film about the rigid control of a psychotic patient in an
American mental hospital, invited his outraged, progressive audience to come forward with offers of care for
the man; there were no takers.)

Conditioning means teaching a new habit at a physiological level. The classical example is that of Pavlov's
dogs who salivated when they heard the dinner bell even
when food wasn't brought. The best-known example is
the bell-and-pad for bed wetting. The first drop of urine
on the metal-grid pad completes a circuit which sounds a
buzzer and the child wakes up. In principle, the sense of
a full bladder about to empty is supposed to become the
stimulus that results in the conditioned response of
waking up. Again, it is a most effective treatment *if* the
child doesn't fiddle with the apparatus, *if* child, family
and therapist make sure the equipment is working, the
procedure understood, and *if* they all persist; which
again illustrates the importance of organisation and
motivation as well as physiological theory if behaviour
therapy is to work.

Response prevention is used for obsessional-compulsive

behaviour, habits the child or adolescent wants to be rid of but can't abandon. A firm and trusted therapist simply does not allow the behaviour, and the young person gradually learns that no disaster follows if he or she doesn't carry out the magically protective habit. An interesting link between behavioural and psychodynamic methods is seen when it is found that the child trusts the therapist to intervene in this way, and the therapist trusts himself to persist with what can be a difficult and anxiety-making technique, but the same mutual confidence may not exist in the child's family. It often then emerges that for improvement to be maintained the family must learn the technique, *and come to terms in some way with the individual or family problems that prevent them confidently and competently implementing it together*. There is no incompatibility between a dual approach of behaviour therapy on the one hand and work with the family dynamics on the other. Together they can be most effective.

Massed practice is a method of extinguishing unwanted habits by insisting that they are carried out to excess. It sometimes works. *Desensitisation* and *flooding* are, respectively, gradual and total exposure, in trusted company, to a feared object or situation.

This short account of behaviour therapy would not be complete without mentioning the diagnostic procedure of *behaviour analysis*. This is a meticulous procedure which assesses the situations in which certain behaviour arises, and it is a point of contact between behavioural treatment and social and family dynamics. Unwanted behaviour may be contingent upon quite subtle environmental factors which might go unnoticed to the inexperienced eye. Why a line of treatment works one day and not the next might be a mystery until it emerges that a child can cope with, say, a peer group of four but misbehaves or panics with five or six. Instructions given by the therapist sitting down in a room with the child may be taken very seriously, but rapidly forgotten if given in less formal circumstances. Treatment carried out by parents may be remarkably effective most of the time, but inexplicably lapse every so often, until it emerges that it depends on which parent is taking the leading part.

Physical treatment

Physical ill health and disability do not have to be very serious in themselves to undermine a child's performance and confidence. The wrong spectacles, or unrecognised hearing impairment or clumsiness, may be as significant as diabetes, asthma or epilepsy. Physical ill health or handicap can affect mood, concentration and social development in general or in quite specific ways, as when unrecognised epilepsy leads to major educational problems. Conversely, chronic ill health, particularly when the disorder is heavily socially stigmatised, again as with epilepsy,[102] can lead to anxiety and despair which in turn results in parents and child coping with the disorder less than competently, either with neglect or too much fuss. Nor are doctors immune to one extreme or the other.

The relationship between emotional problems with physical symptoms, and physical problems with emotional symptoms, is immensely complicated. A child with epilepsy may have epileptic fits that occur for unknown physical reasons; fits due to inefficient medication; real fits provoked by certain emotional states (not necessarily 'stressful'; boredom may do the same); and simulated fits. The most striking example I have seen of the complexity (and strength) of the interaction between the nervous system and psychological and social dynamics was a brain-damaged child whose epilepsy and electroencephalogram (EEG) were worse when he was being fussed over and read to and generally allowed to be passive by his anxious, excessively protective mother.

When the advice she was given by doctors, and the help she was given by her husband, enabled her to be less guilty and to allow the child to take more risks and be more active in big ways and small, his epilepsy and EEG improved on less medication. The advice and support doctors and husband now gave the child's mother directly affected her handling of him, and this in turn directly affected his state of cerebral functioning. The problem was basically physical, but the most effective treatment was marital and psychodynamic therapy and education.

Drugs[93] are an embarrassment to some child psychiatrists who feel that they are abusing a child by prescribing medication, an attitude that may be reinforced by their tending not to see the minority of ill children who need it. This is no accident; selective reinforcement occurs between family doctor and specialist as well as between specialist and patient; the GP soon picks up what sorts of referrals Dr X is none too keen on.

Leaving aside drugs prescribed for physical ill health, including epilepsy, the medication useful to child psychiatrists falls into four broad categories.

1 *Tranquillising and sedating drugs* such as chlorpromazine ('Largactil'), haloperidol ('Serenace') and benzodiazepine drugs such as 'Librium' and 'Valium'. There are many others, some with unwanted side-effects for which it is common to prescribe concurrent medication such as procyclidine ('Kemadrin').

2 *Anti-depressive drugs* such as imipramine ('Tofranil'), amitryptilline ('Tryptizol') and many others.

3 *Lithium carbonate*, a mood-stabilising drug which is effective in manic-depressive illness in adolescents and adults, and may help some disorders in some children and adolescents too.[98] It requires careful monitoring clinically and by regular blood tests.

4 *Central nervous system stimulants*, such as amphet-

amine and methylphenidate, for a small number of children with the hyperkinetic syndrome, an over-diagnosed and imprecisely diagnosed condition.[16]

Drugs can certainly be abused, but child psychiatrists tend to be more enthusiastic about other sorts of treatment.[36] This is all very well but may mean that there may be times and places where no one has much expertise in what medication can do for a minority of very ill children. There is not the slightest doubt that some drugs can help some children and adolescents a great deal. The problem, as with psychotherapy and behaviour therapy, is a) that trouble has to be taken to balance advantages against disadvantages, and b) the other dimensions of treatment must not be neglected. Many practitioners claim to be eclectic, but there is often an insidious slide towards the preferred line of treatment, be it drugs or psychotherapy or whatever, to the detriment of others.

Tranquillising drugs reduce pathological states of arousal – anxiety, excitement or anger – in some highly disturbed children, notably those with psychotic disorders, and so can allow other forms of help (educational, social and psychological) a chance to work. In some disorders, notably some forms of schizophrenia, as arousal levels diminish experiences such as delusions or hallucinations are reduced too.

Anti-depressive drugs are used for depressive disorders in children, but they are also used when a disorder that is not overtly depressive in form is believed to be depressive in nature. Perhaps the simplest example would be a child who has not reacted particularly unhappily to the sudden death of a parent, yet for the next year or two is incapacitated by stomach pains and sleeplessness and poor school performance. He or she may be physically fit, smilingly deny any problem, and be quite unable to benefit from a psychotherapeutic approach, but improve on medication; indeed, improvement may lead on to a more appropriate expression of feelings about her loss, and make psychotherapeutic help feasible.

These drugs may help some bed wetting children, although whether by affecting mood, sleep or the bladder itself is not clear.[94]

All that need be said about lithium and the CNS stimulants has been said above. They are useful for a small minority of children, and, as with many forms of treatment, the precise predictors of a useful response in the cases of individual children are far from clear.

If medication embarrasses some child psychiatrists, the prospect of using *electroconvulsive treatment* (ECT) for children causes anxiety and guilt in most. The controversy, anger and misunderstanding surrounding this treatment need not be elaborated here. It is exceedingly rarely indicated, and then only in children old enough to show adult-type depressive symptoms. If a child goes on and on exhibiting symptoms and signs of profound depression of the sort that, in adults, tends to respond to ECT; if a great deal of distress and handicap is being caused to the child; and if all other treatments, carefully and thoroughly tried, fail to help, I think it should be considered. If so, the reasons for using ECT, the chances of it being helpful, and what it will be like should be discussed with child, family and those who referred the boy or girl in the first place.

Nursing

Like occupational therapy, the nursing profession is so tied to the hospital service that the role of the child psychiatric nurse is often left out when child psychiatric services are discussed. Nursing becomes most relevant when children are admitted to hospital, but the profession is steadily becoming more involved with day-hospital and domiciliary work. Moreover, paediatric nurses have increasingly recognised their need to understand more about the families of children in hospital, and the feelings of the children themselves. A great deal of lip-service has been paid to the emotional needs of families whose children are in hospital, and those of the boys and girls themselves. Individual nurses and teams can do superb work, but the handling of feelings can also be clumsy in the extreme.

The core role of the child psychiatric nurse is hard to define. Clearly the way the profession organises itself enables it to look after children round the clock, every day, and to act in a 'front line' capacity in applying and monitoring psychiatric, psychological and social methods of treatment. But by taking on the demanding task of twenty-four-hour cover, which someone has to do, the profession has fallen behind in clarifying its own individual skills, researching them and teaching them. Instead of consolidating its professional status in the latter ways, it has gone for the wrong option by developing an impressive-looking administrative hierarchy instead, which ambitious and intelligent nurses are supposed to climb once they have spent a few years on the wards. This trend has recently been slightly reversed, probably inadequately.

The special functions of nursing, which differentiate it from other professions, seem to be a) being with the child – awake – day and night; care staff in children's homes of course go to bed; b) applying and monitoring a wide range of treatments; c) being able to care for a child with the skill of the very best child care workers. If a child does not need a) or b), then, in my view, he does not need to be in hospital.[99]

Examples

1   A severely obsessional teenager cannot get out of the house until mid-day in order to complete hand-washing rituals associated with a fear of contaminating other

people with his 'germs'. He knows this is foolish but his tension is so great if he doesn't carry out cleaning rituals to perfection that he repeatedly gives in to them, hoping unrealistically, like an addict, that 'once more' will be enough. The final getting out of the house is a complex business aided by his mother, who opens and closes doors for him, etc. If it goes wrong (or she tries to give up in exasperation) he is enraged and panic-stricken and has to start all over again.

Out-patient psychotherapy and attempts at behaviour therapy fail to help. He is admitted to an adolescent unit, and a behaviour therapy programme planned by a psychologist and implemented by nurses works in a matter of days. The approach does not, however, work at home; the parents cannot summon up the resolve to follow the treatment schedule and cope with the boy's tantrums. It seems that they cannot because of the mutual suspicion and recrimination that develop between the parents whenever they try to get together about anything, and a social worker's gentle but insistent enquiry reveals a major marital problem for which the parents cannot accept help. Although help is refused, it is agreed to acknowledge the problem in a family meeting, and the boy reveals that he suspected it all along. It has been a chronic source of anxiety for him, leading to the bed-time checking and double-checking with which his troubles began years before.

He feels much better now that the matter is out in the open, and the parents are able to patch things up a little. His obsessional habits are improved but not gone, and still interfere with his schoolwork. Ideally, the team would prefer to offer marital therapy, followed by family therapy, in parallel with continuing behaviour therapy for the obsessional symptoms, but the first two are declined. However, the beginning of exploring feelings together has made the boy feel happier about leaving the house, while before he would have been immensely anxious about whether there would be a home to come back to; he is found an ordinary boarding school where his symptoms disappear, he works well academically and develops a better social life.

2   A boy in a children's home threatens another with a knife; he gets very angry because the boy has said he is homosexual, and he threatens to kill him. The staff report that the child seemed 'not himself', 'out of control' when he grabbed the knife, and they believe this to be a manifestation of something quite beyond their normal capacity for care and discipline: the boy seems mad. The visiting child psychiatrist is under great pressure to move the boy to hospital, and his social worker under pressure to move him to more secure accommodation. At an interview, the psychiatrist finds nothing about the boy (such as delusional thinking, a serious mood disorder or a history of aggressive behaviour) that makes a homicidal attack likely; on the other hand he cannot *guarantee* that there is no chance of a similar incident. A talk about some sexual anxieties and misunderstandings the boy has, and his feelings about the parents who abandoned him as puberty approached, seems to relieve his tension.

The boy who provoked him is something of a teaser, and this has led to lesser incidents before: he is made to stop; no one has told him to before. The staff talk over with psychiatrist and social worker the risks (including the professional risks to themselves) of letting the boy stay in the children's home, versus the risks to the boy of having to uproot himself and start again in a hospital or secure unit. The boy is brought into the discussion and asked what he can do to be a bit more predictable; this turns out to include talking over topics the staff have avoided. He doesn't want to see the psychiatrist again, but would like to talk things over regularly with one of the residential staff, who in turn welcomes support and advice from the psychiatrist. The boy settles down; there is a similar but far less threatening incident a month later, with which the staff cope well, and no further problems.

3 A small girl screams and screams and screams at bedtime. Her mother cannot get her to settle. More and more different sorts of sedation are tried but it only makes the girl confused and more upset than ever. Interviews with the parents reveal that the mother had strikingly similar night-time fears and problems, and is still nervous about the dark, especially when her lorry-driver husband is away. A great deal of what seems like useful work is done both in helping the mother in her method of settling her daughter for the night, and in exploring a number of mixed and painful feelings she had about her parents and now about her marriage. Indeed, she and the marriage improve in a number of unanticipated ways, and she is delighted, but *still* the little girl screams and screams at night. Now, however, a very small dose of a sedative drug works, and after a few weeks can be discontinued.

4 A boy has not been to school for over a year, and is described as school phobic. His father wants him to go to school, and leaves this to his wife to handle; she is made miserable by 'pushing' the tearful, frightened boy at the school gates. Father hasn't time to come to the clinic. The Education Department want the boy 'treated' so that he can go back to school. The clinic staff have seen the boy and do not consider that he has a phobic disorder; if he had they would take a behaviour therapy approach, supplemented by medication if the boy was truly panic-stricken. They feel his nervousness about entering an increasingly unfamiliar setting is a combination of his mother's anxiety and the lack of any concerted insistence that as a normal young man he should go to school.

It is pointed out to the Education Department and the family that the clinic can only help if both parents attend regularly; he won't go to school unless both parents insist that he does. The parents however won't do this, and the Education Department decides against taking legal action; they regard the boy as phobic and the clinic as unhelpful. Home tuition is offered by the Education Department instead, despite the psychiatrist's warning that this may comply with the law but won't help the boy, who may well have trouble making friends and, in due course, getting to work.

In fact he does quite well, socially and in the job he eventually gets, although he would have been bright enough for day-release training had he been able to get to college.

5 A psychiatrist is asked to see a girl in a general medical ward. She has taken an overdose of drugs for the sixth or seventh time and comes from a very disturbed family, who often leave her in charge of a large group of much younger children for hours at a time. The general physician wants her out, there being nothing wrong with her. The psychiatrist agrees that she is not suffering from a depressive illness, and agrees that her behaviour is clearly manipulative. Social work reports in her notes give a long history of delinquency and neglect; an attempt to get a care order has been turned down by the magistrates. She is not ill; she *is* quite appropriately attention-seeking, and may very well kill herself whether she wants to or not. She is keen to go into the psychiatric hospital, but when her parents are eventually contacted they say they would discharge her, which they could do since she is under sixteen. The psychiatrist feels she must be away from home, but compulsory admission under a section of the Mental Health Act 1959, even though it would over-ride her parents' wishes, is not appropriate for her mental state, which is not abnormal. The social work department could not feel more strongly that this is absolutely clearly a medical problem, and in any case the only children's home place they have is

inappropriate for a very disturbed girl whose parents are well known for turning up with several large brothers and making a fuss, threatening legal action and so on. Discussions continue late into the night; the medical ward grudgingly agrees to keep her until the morning, by which time it has been agreed to put the girl on a Place of Safety order. She is admitted to the psychiatric hospital for a few days on the understanding that a place in a children's home will be forthcoming next week, and that the psychiatrist will continue to see her as an out-patient.

6   A child has developed normally until the age of nine when he gradually develops poor appetite and sleep, and then begins to have panic attacks and loses interest in his friends, school work and play. Nothing unusual can be found in the way the family operates, and the child's health seems good. Prolonged attempts at individual psychotherapy, using play techniques, reveal only fearfulness and muddle and the child makes no progress, and cannot say what is worrying him, although his drawings reveal a preoccupation with violent incidents and monsters. Psychological testing reveals a significant fall-off in intellectual performance, although he is difficult to assess because of lack of interest in the tests, and high levels of anxiety. A trial of anti-depressants makes him worse, but a small dose of a tranquilliser – chlorpromazine – helps a little. He goes into a prominent paediatric hospital for further physical investigation, one of the rare forms of brain degeneration being feared. The child's parents remember what they have forgotten before, that no less than two distant relatives died early, one with a 'stroke' and the other with multiple sclerosis. Is there any connection? No physical abnormalities are found, despite X-rays, a brain scan, EEG tests and various biochemical tests. Further psychological testing shows no further fall-off in performance. The psychiatrist wonders if this is the early development of a schizo-

phrenic illness, which is particularly rare at this age, or a still more rare degenerative brain disorder. Only a brain biopsy would confirm the latter, and on balance – because of completely normal physical tests so far, and the absence of any treatment for such brain disease – it isn't indicated. All that can be done is to press on trying to establish contact with the child's fears and moods, in order to help him as much as possible, and to look for clinical clues; to keep the family in the picture and cope with the inevitable uncertainty; to organise what schooling and other activities the child can cope with; and to plan to repeat the physical, psychological and EEG testing once or twice a year to see how things develop. Time passes and it is eventually concluded that the child has developed schizophrenia, and although chlorpromazine and special schooling keep him moderately relaxed and contented, the rest of the family's loss is real, and the social worker seeing them regularly helps them with what is, in effect, grief.

7   A teenage boy is referred as '? psychotic' to the psychiatric clinic. It emerges that he has been drawing very bizarre and sexually sadistic pictures in his school books and misbehaving. 'He isn't the nice boy he used to be.' Everyone at school and at home is very alarmed. It emerges that the boy is less bright than the teachers thought, his liveliness and imaginativeness hiding the fact that his intellectual level, after careful testing, is only a little above the level known as 'educationally subnormal' – ESN. His family is a kind, well-meaning, rather chaotic one, and problems have tended to be mocked and laughed off, not without success, so far. One by one the children have left home more or less successfully, but big sister has just left under a cloud, going off with the man who got her pregnant. The parents, themselves emotionally rather immature, with no friends and little social life, and both with a background of family problems, do not know how to cope

with their disappointment with advancing years and with their son's and their daughter's behaviour.

The psychiatrist is satisfied that the boy's only problems are his emotional immaturity, relatively low intelligence and chaotic and really rather unhappy family. With only one of these problems, or perhaps even two, he would never have come to psychiatric attention, but the combination of all three tips the balance. The psychiatrist and psychologist see the family together for a few sessions, helping them talk over ordinary disappointments and fears they haven't talked over before, and where the boy needs limits more firmly set on his behaviour the parents are cajoled and encouraged into taking a firmer line. For the first time they are persuaded to go along to talk over their son's behaviour with the head teacher – they felt nervous and inhibited about doing so before – and the psychologist goes along with them by way of support. The whole business has a sobering effect on the young man, and he feels a good deal more secure, sufficiently so to talk sensibly about trying to get a job, although there isn't one to be had. Fortunately he is found a place at an industrial training centre; how well he will maintain his improvement, and the family their new-found confidence, if he cannot get a job is another matter.

8 A child psychiatrist refers a child back to a social work department as unsuitable for psychotherapy; the latter was tried and failed. The social worker learns that the child's attendance was erratic, he saw the psychiatrist on some occasions and his assistant on others, and some sessions seemed to have lasted about twenty minutes. The social worker has no idea whether this is true, nor whether the psychiatrist has special expertise in psychotherapy. He is advised by his senior that he had better accept the psychiatrist's opinion, because relationships with that clinic are rather strained at the moment, and they have another child to refer.

The organisation and management of treatment

It will be clear from the above account of different approaches to treatment that for the most part they cannot be carried out by the psychiatrist simply sitting in his room with the child, although this is how many people imagine a psychiatrist works. Certainly a limited amount can be done in this way, and perhaps individual psychotherapy with an adolescent who is looking after himself at home and school (or work) is the best example.

But for most children, in diagnosis, in managing treatment and monitoring progress, other work has to be done too.

First, to return to an earlier theme, all children need education, care and control. The psychiatrist isn't trained to provide this, even if he had the time and the inclination. The psychiatrist has to make sure that if he is going to take on treatment, someone else is going to look after the child, get him up in the morning, feed him properly, get him to school and so on. In many cases no special attention has to be paid to school, other than obtaining occasional progress reports from teachers and being available to them if needed. But it is most unusual for the rest of the family not to need advice, or explanation, or support, or occasionally one of the therapies. (The exception, in my view, is the older adolescent leading a genuinely independent and more or less competent life who refers himself or herself for individual help.) For the psychiatrist not to pay close attention to the background of the child he is treating would be like another doctor prescribing vitamin pills for malnutrition, or binding up cuts and breakages week after week, without trying to deal with the way they arise.

Second, some treatment with some children is far

more appropriately carried on by someone closer to the child in an ordinary, non-clinical sense. If a child needs help with organising his life, affection more clearly and unequivocally expressed in his family, limits set consistently and firmly, fears and fantasies aired and dealt with, it is far better if the child's teachers or parents or both do this, all week, than for the psychiatrist to do it on a sessional basis. Usually the non-clinical adults will have some good ideas too; they will certainly know things about the family's and school's strengths that the psychiatrist will not know of. Just because the child has been referred to the psychiatrist doesn't mean that everyone else is necessarily feeling helpless. And if they are, there is work to be done there too.

Third, the range of work is too wide for the psychiatrist to be sufficiently competent at all of it; and even in those areas where he can be, he would not have the time to do it all unless he treated only a handful of patients a week. The role of the child psychiatrist is a key theme in chapter 7. For the moment, having already distinguished *treatment* from *care*, education (training) and *control*, I would subdivide *treatment* further into:

(a) That requiring the skills of general medical practice and clinical psychiatry, the latter including the skill of assessing and monitoring mental functioning, mood, ideas and beliefs.

(b) Psychotherapeutic skills, including expertise in understanding and handling relationships, primarily verbally, or primarily *via* active and creative techniques.

(c) Skills in social administration: knowing what is available where, in the way of special resources, and how to organise it, fill in the right forms and so on.

(d) Skill in measuring mental functioning, particularly reasoning and learning ability, in a standardised way.

(e)   Skill in organising the behaviour of the child and others in order to encourage some patterns of behaviour and discourage others.

At the risk of upsetting professional workers who see their skills quite differently, I am suggesting that most psychiatrists are best at (a); social workers, psychotherapists, 'social therapists', different sorts of creative and occupational therapists and family therapists best at (b); social workers also adept at (c); psychologists best at (d) and (e). Of course these fields overlap, and for example you will find psychologists and psychiatrists prominent among leading psychotherapists. But an individual professional worker is characteristically very good in one area, quite good in another, able to get by in a third, and not much use elsewhere. Yet the child and family presenting at a psychiatric clinic with an as yet undiagnosed problem are entitled to expect skills to be available in this whole range, *and* for them to be used judiciously, *and* for the clinic staff to be able to recognise needs that they cannot meet, but to know where to look for them.

They are also entitled to expect that the staff will give them all the time they need, yet not to have too long a waiting list; and to be the sort of people who have a timetable that allows them time to keep up to date in a range of complicated and developing fields. They will also expect a firm and confident enough approach, but that areas of doubt will be expressed honestly – that they will be told the truth. They will presumably expect good organisation, and that someone will be in charge, responsible for the way they are treated, supervising the less experienced staff; yet not in the style of a rigid, bureaucratic, autocratic machine. Finally (for they are optimists) they would hope for similar qualities among the staff of other facilities and departments whose co-operation the clinic team may need to enlist.

All this is quite a tall order, and one that is not

universally met, in child psychiatry or in other areas of child care.

Conclusions

The various professionals concerned with disturbed children have developed a wide range of quite different sorts of treatment. They are all difficult to apply well, needing careful monitoring (and supervision for all but the most experienced staff) as well as initial training. Moreover, as earlier chapters showed, it is far from clear which children need which treatment, and which need any treatment at all, although out of a well-meaning and to some extent inevitable muddle, some very troubled children and their families get a good deal of excellent help.

At the heart of the matter there are some definite enough problems, and a number of useful treatments. But clarifying the problems and selecting and implementing treatment is a complicated task, partly because a great deal remains unclear about psychiatric disorder, but also because a good deal of the uncertainty and complexity extends well beyond clinical work and into matters of ethics, philosophy, law and social policy. Finally, organising what a child needs can be very difficult.

One of the axioms of the age is that people with psychiatric disorder (as well as having nothing wrong with them) are incurable; that psychiatric treatment is often ineffective. An important aspect of that tendency to ineffectiveness has nothing to do with lack of knowledge or the 'mystery of the mind', but the difficulty inherent in organising psychiatric work, and in particular in the problems professionals meet in working together in this field. We have already seen how many different sorts of approaches there are to treatment; in the whole child care, treatment and educational field there are a range of philosophies, methods and facilities, determined not so much by need as by the way different professions have developed. The next chapter briefly outlines some aspects of this history, and then chapter 7 looks at the issues that arise when people try to work together in the interests of children.

6

The Development of Services for Children

There was an old woman who lived in a shoe
She had so many children she didn't know what to do
She gave them some broth, without any bread,
And whipped them all soundly and sent them to bed.

The problem of the old lady in the shoe has been recorded in the traditional nursery rhyme for 200 years, but uncertainty about what we do with children, especially difficult children, and especially in the up-bringing of other people's children (to use Tizard's phrase)[105] goes back well before then. In less complex, more slowly changing cultures, often with a high infant mortality taken for granted, the survivors grew up and played until, on a specific day, they underwent a ritual that acknowledged that they were now adults, fit to work and bring up their own children. In the Middle Ages, at least in Western cultures, children were not acknowledged as individual people with rights and needs; they were infants until the age of seven or eight, and then small adults. A protracted middle childhood and adolescence as a significant period of life is a relatively recent concept. Only in the last hundred or so years, with more to learn and train for in order to take part in adult life, has the idea – if not the practice – of a prolonged and proper preparation for adult life become widespread.[27] Indeed, it has been taken to extremes in professional circles, where men and women well into their thirties and forties continue to be in training, being supervised and taking examinations; this is a situation not without its significance for child care and child psychiatry, where troubled children are often being looked after by people who are not sure that they are quite adult.

As children were taken more seriously, because of industrial needs and perhaps because of a growing awareness by influential adults of children's needs, rights and feelings, the professions concerned with teaching and looking after other people's children began to emerge. Previously the churches had been largely responsible for education, except in Greece and Rome. Broadly speaking, six facets of individual children's qualities and attributes became important for one reason or another: their social background – prince or pauper; their behaviour, largely in terms of their obedience; their educational achievements in the widest sense, such as ability to play, read, sing and work; their ability to learn what adults wanted to teach them; their physical health; and their sanity.

In different periods and circumstances different aspects would receive attention. Extremes of imbecility or madness would be noticed, though often confused with each other, as they often are to this day. Physical weakness, illness and death might be variously important to a family, to the employer of child labour, and occasionally to the legal authorities. Lesser degrees of physical or mental handicap would be important for people setting themselves up to educate children. Different sorts of children were recognised: good children, bad children, dull children, possessed children, wicked children, abandoned children, idiot children, insane children, nervous children, delinquent children and remarkable children. There has been something for them all, although what this has been has varied enormously and has sometimes been appalling. In response to the problems, behaviour or perceived needs of groups of children over the centuries a whole range of variegated adult responses developed, some of them becoming institutionalised and turning into the various child training, treatment and care professions. Child psychiatry, its role blurred at the edges, both gaining from and contributing to related fields, has been consistently associated with developments in these professions. Its relationship to them has been sometimes central, sometimes peripheral and often ambiguous, so that many of the public can even now hardly tell child psychiatrists, psychologists, educationalists, sociologists and criminologists apart, nor for that matter the work they do.

Control, punishment and education

Considering that children are the human race's most important production and most valuable asset, the way they have been handled by their elders is astonishing and sometimes horrifying. Moments of enlightenment have occurred however, even if you look back a long way. For example, King Athelstan (924–39 AD), King Alfred's grandson, introduced an alternative to the execution of misbehaving boys, who were put on a form of probation instead, if their families wouldn't take responsibility for them. However, if the boy persisted in his misdemeanours he was killed.[15,66] Judicial child killing continued until relatively recently in this country. As late as 1831 a boy of nine was hanged at Chelmsford for fire-setting.[45]

Both misuse of children and measures to protect them often centred on their use in the labour market. The medieval guilds, for example, not necessarily always primarily for humane reasons, provided employment and training for children and regulated hours of work. In the time of Henry VIII there was growing concern at the large numbers of vagrant children, and all those between five and fourteen were made liable to be bound over to a master as apprentices, the boys until twenty-four, and the girls until twenty. In 1601 a statute was passed which enabled not only the children of vagrants and orphans to be apprenticed, but also the children of those parents who were burdened with them and unable to support them. In the industrial revolution at the end of the eighteenth century one route for children was into the mills, and it is interesting that bargains were often struck between parish authorities and mill owners to take one mentally retarded child with every twenty; many of these children disappeared. Millham and his colleagues[66] have described vividly how from the early seventeenth century onwards large numbers of children were transported or sent to sea; Hansard in 1891 recorded a plea for boys to replace the 4000–5000 sailors drowned yearly in the Mercantile Marine.

During the nineteenth century institutions for the criminal, the ill and the poor grew, paralleled by a vast expansion in boarding school education. Throughout, the response to troublesome children, when not purely punitive, was to put them in an institution.

An 1896 report, however, not only stressed the need for care rather than punishment, but questioned whether offending children should be removed from home and placed with large numbers of other delinquents. The debate continues with such recent developments as the Children and Young Persons Act, 1969, which moved the emphasis of dealing with difficult children from the courts to the social services, family therapy, and experimental schemes such as those in Kent to place children who cannot remain in their own family with another.[40]

Developments over the centuries have led to a wide range of assorted establishments, uneasily balancing care, education and control: Community Homes with Education (descended from the approved schools); remand, assessment and reception centres; secure units[66] detention centres (including those with 'short, sharp shock' facilities), and borstals; a wide range of children's homes and hostels run by local authorities or independent organisations, some of them well known charities; and a variety of therapeutic communities and special boarding schools.

Education has its own complex history. It emerges here partly because of the necessity for educating institutionalised children, once the law of the land required it, and also because of its relationship with developments in psychology and certain approaches to therapy.

It is difficult to be sure of all the motives and aims of the adults involved in planning and running the above institutions. Undoubtedly they were mixed, and concepts of punishment, containment and control would have been mixed to varying degrees with concern about children and their welfare and the wish to train them to the moral and ethical standards of the day.

With the spread of the state's interest in education, and later the introduction of compulsory education in Europe in the eighteenth and nineteenth centuries and parallel with the burgeoning of the new science of psychology, the idea gained ground that the understanding, sorting-out and management of children (as well as adults) might now be based on more than just *ad hoc* expediency and common sense. Important developments whose consequences are still with us took place at around the same time; around the turn of the century Sigmund Freud was publishing and lecturing in the new field of psychoanalysis, in 1905 Binet and Simon devised the first intelligence test, and in 1906 Pavlov reported the results of his studies on the conditioning of behaviour.

In England, centres were being established which took the anthropological and biological approach to mental life which had been developed by Charles Darwin and Francis Galton; in 1893 Sully established the British Child Study Association, the object of which was to help teachers cope with children's problems by using psychological, social and anthropometric methods.[107] Meanwhile, implementation of the Elementary Education Act 1870, and its statutory successors, was revealing differences in children's capacity to respond to teaching, and led to the London County Council appointing its own psychologist, Cyril Burt, in 1913.

All these growing points in the fields of dynamic psychology, the measurement of intellect and aptitude, and behavioural psychology, are still proliferating, and the descendants of these early workers are to be found among specialist teachers, child and family psychiatrists and psychotherapists, and academic clinical and educational psychologists. Whatever proportion of the numerous institutions mentioned earlier actually have members of one or more of these professions on their staff, it certainly seems the norm now that they should. To an important extent, however, the introduction of these new approaches to children took place in special therapeutic schools, notably pioneered by Maria Montessori in 1898 in Rome, and Rudolf Steiner in 1919 in Stuttgart.

The origins of the child guidance clinics and child psychiatry

At around this time the first moves were being made to establish clinics for children with emotional, social and educational problems.

It is interesting to reflect for a moment that clinic means bed; at least *klinikos* does in Greek. Clinical is a medical term *par excellence* with intimations of the sick-bed, the bedside manner, and so on. Be that as it may, clinics they were called when the first centres for helping children in difficulties by psychological and psychiatric means got off the ground.

Montessori, a medical doctor, may have been among the first in the field when she took a special interest in

the problems of children in her psychiatric clinic at the
University of Rome from about 1904. The first organised
clinic for children was Healey's Chicago Juvenile Psy-
chopathic Unit, opened in 1909 for delinquents and
staffed by what was to become irreverently known as the
'holy trinity' of psychiatrist, psychologist and social
worker. In 1917 the Judge Baker Guidance Centre began
in Boston and in 1921 Thoms set up the Boston Habit
Clinic.[107] In England the Tavistock Clinic had been
treating children since 1926, the East London Child
Guidance Clinic was established under the direction of
Dr Emanuel Miller in 1927, and the London Child
Guidance Clinic was opened in 1936 as a treatment and
training clinic, directed by Dr William Moody. By then,
there was a Child Guidance Council, and by 1937 it had
recognised forty-six clinics.

Social workers were taking an active part in establish-
ing and staffing these new clinics. Emerging initially as
voluntary workers with independent and charitable
organisations, they were by now becoming established
in a profession with training and qualifications.[31, 59] By
now there were many varieties of social and welfare
worker including the medical social worker whose for-
bear, the hospital almoner, had originally had the task of
assessing the financial state of patients. Social work is
now an elaborately organised and large profession and
its role controversial.[5, 75]

Hospital child psychiatry

The early history of mental hospitals includes scattered
references to young people regarded as 'mentally defective' or 'mentally deranged' and occasional, individual
case reports such as that of the 'wild boy' of Aveyron.[48, 70] Mentally retarded children were noted in
the records of workhouses, public infirmaries and
asylums, but in general children received little mention
in the early history of institutional psychiatry, although

we can assume that mentally ill young people were put in asylums from time to time. There certainly seemed a demand to be met, because by the end of the Maudsley Hospital's first year of functioning, in 1924, it had treated forty-four patients under fourteen years of age, of whom eight had been admitted.[107]

Meanwhile, general hospitals had begun to provide special provision for sick children from the middle of the nineteenth century, and as these departments developed, psychiatrists began to appear on their staff. While delinquents were getting what society considered their just deserts, for example, in the prison hulks in the estuaries of large cities,[66] the hospitals were providing wards for acute illness and country convalescent homes for large numbers of poor children convalescing from infectious diseases.

By the 1930s experience of children as in-patients in psychiatric units was beginning to build up, especially in America, prompted in the 1920s by the need for provision for children suffering from the after-effects of epidemic encephalitis.[1] The first psychiatric hospital out-patient clinic for children in this country began operating at the Maudsley Hospital in 1939, its in-patient unit, initially at Mill Hill, opening the following year. The first psychiatric unit for adolescents in this country was opened at St Ebba's Hospital in 1948, moving later to Long Grove Hospital, and in 1949 the Adolescent Unit at Bethlem Royal Hospital was opened.[107] Both hospitals took 'voluntary' patients, this being the exception rather than the rule at that time, and perhaps partly for this reason had already accumulated adolescents in their adult wards.

In the last thirty years many more children's and adolescents' in-patient units have appeared all over the country, Barker's book on the subject appearing in 1974, listing seventy-four.[1] More, it is frequently said, are needed.[25]

Other special centres

Various secure units and special schools have already been mentioned. In addition there are some well known therapeutic communities for young people, such as Peper Harow and the Cotswold Community. There are also a very few special centres for autistic children, and some therapeutic homes and hostels for children and older adolescents, for example those run on Rudolf Steiner principles and by the Richmond Fellowship. There are also advisory services and walk-in clinics, such as the Brent Consultation Centre in London; units dealing with, among other problems, child abuse;[60] paediatric clinics run in liaison with child psychiatrists; day hospitals and day centres for children with either a psychiatric or an educational emphasis; state and independent homes for the mentally handicapped, and of course psychiatrists, psychologists and others working privately.

Organisations

This diversity is reflected in the many organisations and journals dealing with this field. Characteristically, in professional training, there is hardly the time or the opportunity to become acquainted with more than just the few more closely related to one's own field of work. There are numerous professional, educational, self-help and pressure groups too, dealing with all the common forms of problem and handicap, and these also have their publications. The best way for the newcomer to the subject to find out about organisations and publications outside his or her immediate professional preoccupation is with the help of specialist librarians, while the bibliographies of useful articles and books will provide guidance too.

The field today

Chapter 3 ended with the point that in the course of a year some 5–15 per cent of children and adolescents have problems which could be regarded as psychiatric, depending of course on how the problem was defined. One could take 10 per cent as a rough guide, bearing in mind that the incidence of real mental illness is far lower (see chapter 4) while if all the disadvantaged and delinquent children in the country were to be included with those needing some form of special psychological, social or educational help, the number would be far higher, particularly in some inner city areas.[86]

On the one hand, as chapters 3 and 4 showed, there are many thousands of children and adolescents with for the most part rather ill-defined problems, from the relatively trivial to the most severe; on the other hand, there are large numbers of professional workers of very different persuasions, extremely diverse in their training, attitudes, the way they work and the settings in which they operate.

Moreover, the whole field is undergoing change and development. For good or ill, there is considerable experimentation (for example) in education, and psychiatric practice, particularly in child psychiatry, is changing rapidly. In all professional fields an enormous amount is published each year, a good deal of it without lasting value, but nonetheless requiring the attention of the conscientious professional. There is also a great deal of dispute and uncertainty, not merely about diagnosis and treatment, but about the sort of services we need, and where scarce resources should go. There is less money available, but most services, whether social, psychiatric, psychological or educational are inclined to feel they need more in order to do their work properly.

More specifically, there is at the moment a great deal of controversy about the function and leadership of the child guidance clinics, and their relationship to social, educational and psychological services, and indeed to hospital-based child psychiatry.[108] The marriage – or *ménage à trois* – between psychiatrist, psychologist and social worker which raised such high and even utopian hopes in the 1920s has not worked out; the participants are unhappy and many wanting separation.

Psychology has become an independent profession with an uneasy relationship with psychiatry, especially where practising the various psychotherapies is concerned; psychiatrists, psychologists and social workers can each make good cases for this to be their province, rather than that of the other two, with the psychiatric case perhaps the weakest. And yet many of the general public, and quite a lot of psychiatrists too, regard psychotherapy in one form or another as psychiatry's main function.

In a wider perspective, treatments favoured by some are attacked as useless or even harmful by others. Professionalism itself is a term of abuse in some radical-sociological circles, and regarded by them as merely the latest way in which the comfortable middle classes do good, salve their consciences, earn good salaries and maintain the *status quo*. Conversely, the more conservatively inclined see in their critics not a desire to improve on present arrangements, but a wish to undermine anything at all which maintains the existing culture. The various 'children's lib' movements, if they went as far as their proponents wish, would undoubtedly bring about fundamental changes in the way society is organised, since the encouragement of children and adolescents to be deeply suspicious of all adult authority, and to organise themselves to challenge it, would be profoundly undermining of all age groups. Conversely, genuine moves to protect and enhance children's legal rights and protection become tainted with the suspicion that the children's liberators, after the revolution, would soon have boys and girls re-organised into uniformed ranks, singing the party songs. Bringing politics into questions of child care is certainly rather awkward; nevertheless there are fundamental conflicts of belief about how society should be organised, particularly among the professional groups looking after children, and they can only be ignored at the cost of causing unease and discomfort between people who are trying to work together. Indeed, they may be quite comfortable discussing traditionally difficult topics, such as sexual behaviour, but keep cautiously away from potentially divisive issues like the power and pay of different professional groups, the pros and cons of selective and private schooling, attitudes to the police, delinquency and law and order generally, and matters of sex role and private morality. I am not suggesting that professional workers should have moral and political discussion groups; but private beliefs *do* intrude upon decisions made about children, and people should feel reasonably comfortable about them, and able to acknowledge differences of conviction.

A case conference is discussing the considerable progress an adolescent girl is making. Among many problems there has been a marked rebellious streak and uncertainty about her sexual identity. A middle-aged careers adviser (tweed jacket, leather patches, grey flannels) tells the group she stands a higher chance of getting a job now that she has dropped her punk appearance and is beginning to adopt an attractive and feminine appearance and a more deferential manner, and this should be encouraged by her social worker. The radicals in the group go pink and exchange glances, and the liberals feel uncomfortable. Serious discussion about how to help this girl's muddled sense of role and self-esteem is shelved for the moment.

In a wider perspective, the adult world, particularly in Western developed countries, is far from sure about a whole range of ethical and moral issues, and there are mixed feelings in particular about adult authority, and at what age a child should be able to make up his or her own mind and discount parental wishes. Again, as mentioned earlier, many adults find their instinctive feelings on such matters clouded by a suspicion that many powerful cases being made in one direction or another are not directly in the interests of the children, but in pursuit of wider convictions that the community should stay much the way it is, or, alternatively, change radically. Of course it has always been this way; but more people, particularly the modern, middle-class professionals of vaguely liberal inclinations, are now particularly aware of such problems, and perhaps particularly conscious these days that a cosy middle-of-the-road position is going to be increasingly hard to maintain and that hard decisions are going to have to be made about social policy and individual morality that directly affect work with children and with colleagues.

Finally, there are many aspects of professional and inter-professional organisation that militate against good work being done. Menzies[63, 64] has pointed out how professions can actually organise themselves so as to avoid the difficulties inherent in doing the most important and difficult parts of their work.

An excellent psychiatric nurse, seconded to a most prestigious general teaching hospital's obstetrics department as part of her training, got a black mark on her report for 'spending too much time talking to patients'. This was conveyed as evidence of being a poor nurse; the matter of getting the balance right between talking to patients and other duties had not been taken up as a teaching issue.

The implementation of the Salmon Report on the organisation of the nursing profession, and the Seebohm Report on social work, intended to enhance the efficiency and status of these respective professional workers, has resulted in a high-speed flow of the more competent and efficient staff up the professional ladder and into administration. People closest to children stay for a short time in their posts, and are increasingly young and inexperienced. The stoicism of some disturbed children as their individual 'field' workers flit by faster even than the child is moved from home to home is to be admired; it must remind them very much of how their parents behaved before they were taken 'into care', although the reasons for adult lack of genuine interest (which is what it is) among professionals sound far more respectable than the reasons their less articulate parents were able to give.

Meanwhile, the need and demand for training, taking part in educational courses, and 'communicating' with other people in the professional hierarchy and with other professions, together with a reduction in working hours – all necessary and laudable – mean that many professional workers (except those who have given up)[35, 61, 103] operate at a brisk trot, squeezing children and parents into the narrowing gaps left between meetings, support groups and meals. And as each group gets busier, it looks for new sub- and ancillary grades to keep an eye on the kids.

Not all workers however are favoured with lots of teaching and supervision meetings and allowed attendance at policy-making committees. For at the other extreme there are many areas where people doing the most difficult work, such as residential child care workers with disturbed children, have the least training, supervision, support, status, pay and prospects. Nursing staff, dealing face-to-face with children and adolescents too demanding and difficult to manage in children's homes, are in general little better off. Mobility, then, is not always upwards into administration, but out of the child care and treatment field altogether, or into one of the many alternative special therapies that abound. For a large number of people in these fields, the task in hand is to cope and survive in the job; actually enjoying it is for the minority.

Conclusions

Just how much the specialist child care professions have taken on is only now dawning on them. The expensive super-specialists like child psychiatrists, previously lavishing time-consuming and uncertain treatments on a minority of uncertainly selected children, are now putting their houses in order and looking again at their proper roles, leaving the care, control and to a lesser extent the teaching and training professions wondering about what they are going to do with all the children revealed as having primarily social problems. Parents, too, have tended to withdraw or been withdrawn; the experts, even adolescent experts with a degree and a diploma, now know more than they do. And just as the problems inherent in all this are becoming clear, which they are, the money for putting it right, like time, is running out.

What do these children need in the professionals looking after them? Among other things, patience, consistency, sustained affection and interest; mature, confident, secure adults who are skilled and experienced in their jobs, who trust and encourage each other, and who enjoy their lives and work.

7

Problems for Professionals;
Working Together;
Consultation as a
Style of Work

> The planning and development of an integrated
> health service must therefore be done in such a way as
> to facilitate at every level the closest possible working
> relations with these [educational and social] services.
> *Fit for the Future*: the Report on
> Child Health Services, 1976.[25]

But in what way? This slightly ambiguous quotation
gets very close to the heart of the problem. Should the
means by which services are developed include close
attention to those things that get in the way of effective
co-operation between disciplines? Or should the *end
result* be a utopia in which, somehow, people have
been organised into a position where 'the closest
possible working relations' follow automatically? The
latter is probably what is meant.

Professor Court's report, *Fit for the Future*, was a
most thorough and conscientious study of problems and
needs in the field of child health, and while child
psychiatry received a great deal of attention, the role of
child psychiatry was not its prime focus. It is mentioned
here partly because people concerned about services for

children should read it, and partly because in its emphasis on integrating professionals and services, on preventative work, health education and a shift towards health care taking place in the home, the school and the family doctor's surgery, it raises the sort of problematic issues discussed here in earlier chapters. (Disappointingly, the report also recommends the establishment of three new sorts of child care specialist.) It also sees the need for more child psychiatrists and psychiatric units, the integration of child guidance clinics and hospital-based child psychiatry into a single service, for improved services for the chronically psychiatrically ill child and the mentally handicapped, more consultative support provided from psychiatric teams, and for monitoring of new services' effectiveness.

Problems and issues: an outline

To bring together the threads of what has been said so far, and the theme of this chapter, I would like to state the fundamental problems of using child psychiatry as briefly as possible:

1   *The role of child psychiatry* The proper role of child and adolescent psychiatry within the broader context of looking after children is neither clear nor generally agreed.
2   *The referral process* It follows that there is uncertainty and disagreement about when child psychiatrists should be approached, and how they should respond. This uncertainty exists on both sides – within child psychiatry and without.
3   *Questions of competence, authority and training* It also follows that there is a good deal of competition within child psychiatry and outside about who knows best, who should make decisions, what sort of training and career to go for if someone wants to help and work with 'disturbed children', and where priorities should lie for research and teaching.

4 *The complexity of the subject* Although special forms of care and education and even psychotherapy can be practised along reasonably straightforward theoretical lines, this is not true of child psychiatry, where the referral is made because the 'problem' has failed to respond to ordinary measures, or is not understandable in ordinary terms. As has been shown, once resort has been made to child psychiatry, adequate diagnosis of the child and situation requires consideration of social, family, psychological, developmental and physical factors, and their interaction with each other over time. Ability to make sense of the child's problem in such terms requires collaboration between specialists able to understand them, *and* at least a nodding acquaintance with each other's terminology. But the problems are not only conceptual; many legal and ethical dilemmas occur too.

5 *Difficulties inherent in day-to-day work with disturbed children* There are many dilemmas, but, as Eisenberg[28] has pointed out, there is also a need to take action and make decisions, not only in the face of ethical conflict and disagreement, but despite uncertainty about diagnosis, treatment and the risks of acting *versus* not acting. 'First do no harm' is a sound medical dictum, sometimes supporting masterly inactivity; but in child psychiatry, with the child surrounded by anxious adults pressing for different solutions, and with childhood going by, even to take no action requires a definite decision.

In summary, the nature of children's problems makes good collaboration between adults essential; indeed, child psychiatric treatment largely consists of skilled collaboration. And yet, for the reasons that have been given, good collaboration is difficult.

1 The role of child and adolescent psychiatry

It is up to child psychiatrists to state clearly and un-equivocally what they should do, and for whom. This need not be a rigid statement; all healthily operating and developing professions must have room for innovators and people who want to work in different ways. But for the sake of other professions' functioning, for the children and parents who may come psychiatry's way, and for training needs within psychiatry itself, there is a need for a reasonably clear focus for the specialty. An appointments committee, a local community or a general practitioner (to take three perspectives) know pretty well what they are going to get if they are looking for an obstetrician, a policeman or a clergyman. Why should it be different as far as child psychiatrists are concerned?

The uses of child psychiatry and its proper function are the subject of chapter 8, and will not be elaborated here.

2 The referral process

The process by which professional help is sought has received too little attention. This is particularly un-fortunate for child psychiatry (and its clientele) because in few other fields of work is the *concept of disorder* so thoroughly bound up in the *process of referral*, in which I include the preliminaries of a parent or non-psychiatric professional beginning to feel he or she cannot manage, and beginning to wonder if the right person to approach might be a psychiatrist.

This point cannot be over-emphasised. As discussed in chapters 3 and 4, a problem, whether psychological, physical or developmental, can be contained largely 'within' the individual child, whether as a prevailing pattern of ideas and feelings or as an abnormal way of functioning at an anatomical or physiological level. But many children who become psychiatric patients are no different in any way from large numbers of children with other problems or with no problems at all. Their psychiatric status lies entirely in the decision made by adults that they cannot cope with them and that perhaps a psychiatrist can.

Now it could be argued that the same applies to many medical patients. There are many people with hay fever, peptic ulcers, hypertension, rheumatic disorders and varicose veins who never become patients, just as there are people with medical patient status with nothing wrong with them at all. But psychiatric status does carry a stigma, particularly when the very child who gets into psychiatric care in this particular way is the very sort of child most at risk from losing parents, friends, school and other aspects of normal life. This point was made in chapter 2. Children in such states of social *extremis* have very nearly lost everything, which may sound dramatic but is frequently the case nonetheless. In their anxiety, uncertainty and despair everyone involved focuses on psychiatry, into which it is hoped the disturbed child might disappear, to re-emerge different (i.e. cured) when everyone would be only too pleased and able to love and teach and care for them again.

There are two fundamentally different components to the wish for a boy or girl to be seen by a psychiatrist. First, there is a more or less rational hope that the psychiatrist will have a technical method (a treatment) to put the child right.

Second, there is a wish *in the person making the referral* for assistance for himself. I do not want to make too much of this; I am not talking about a 'cry for help' on the part of the referrer, although that may be there. If a parent feels he or she cannot parent enough to help their child's fears or sadness or habits or behaviour, there will be at least a little anxiety and guilt around, some muddled and elusive feelings about failing, and seeking someone else's help; this may be minimal, perhaps microscopic, while at other times it will get in the way of making rational decisions and helping the child appropriately. There are similar feelings around, great or small, if a teacher finds he cannot cope, or if a social worker, psychologist or psychiatrist, called in as the helper *par excellence*, cannot help enough.

The effect of such feelings, which are normal and to an extent inevitable, is potentially damaging: the child is labelled as disturbed, or *very* disturbed; the adult feels pangs of guilt and helplessness which can undermine areas of his or her work which in fact *are* effective, even with that particular child; and then adults, parents and professionals begin to blame each other, a blame which may well not be expressed but be around as a niggly and confidence-sapping feeling that one's seniors, peers, or juniors are not good, or unsupportive, or the school's no good, or the Head's no good, the children's home's no good, and so on. Such feelings, *because* they tend to be muddled and mixed up with anxiety about being too intrusive, too demanding, too critical, too long-suffering, too lax and uncritical, or too discourteous, prevent cool and sensible conclusions being reached about who has the wit and strength and resources to do what. When people say that children are 'driving them mad' they do not always realise how near the truth this is, and how strong and irrational are the feelings evoked when children don't or won't develop in the way expected.

So there are irrational feelings contained in the act of resorting to psychiatric help for a child for whom one is responsible, and this should be understood and acknowledged by referrer and by the psychiatric team. There are irrational feelings, too, in being asked to help, and the professionals on the receiving end should be aware of them.

A child psychiatrist, community physician and family doctor make a joint referral of a mentally retarded boy to another child psychiatrist. The parents, unhappy about a home for handicapped children that has been found for their son, want a 'second opinion'. The child psychiatrist is flattered and arranges the child's admission for further assessment and investigation. The parents' hopes are high, and the three doctors involved in the referral, quite well-informed people within their own fields, really do not know what wonders of recent developments in diagnosis and treatment might be available, or at least just around the corner, in this branch of psychiatry. The parents are immensely grateful to this new doctor on the scene, 'the first one to *really* understand'; he glows within; such accolades aren't too common in this sphere. Detailed investigations come to nothing, although the child improves somewhat because of the good *care, education and control* the hospital, albeit expensively, can provide. The parents' gratitude knows no bounds. Then comes the time for discharge; the boy becomes frightened and regresses, and all hell breaks loose, with the parents' worry, disappointment, guilt and anger, present from the child's birth and the lack of help they received from every professional they approached, all now going in the child psychiatrist's direction.

The parents' feelings, the referring doctors' feelings and indeed the receiving child psychiatrist's feelings are quite genuine and appropriate as feelings go, but they have not been conscious enough for scrutiny and for testing out against harsh reality. Anxious to do something, the professionals have led each other and the family unwittingly up the garden path, and meanwhile the place at the residential home has been lost. Scraping through the piles of notes the child psychiatrist finds enough electro-encephalographic (brain-wave) abnormality to justify the boy's referral to a neurologist, 'just in case'.

When A refers someone to B, whatever their respective roles, contained within the referral should be acceptance in both sides that B need not be expected to take over, but rather that together A and B should explore how A can continue, and what sort of help is needed from B to enable him to do so.

This is the approach taken by Bruggen,[13] and referred to earlier; his team at the Adolescent Unit at Hill End refuses to use medical authority for admission, but instead expects those making the referral to examine why they cannot cope, and what help is needed to enable them to cope. Acceptance that for the moment they cannot cope is regarded as reasonable grounds for a brief admission of the adolescent while the referring agents, including the family, get themselves together again to carry on with the boy or girl. This approach does not meet everyone's needs, but it is an important way of looking at the process by which young people are selected for admission to psychiatric units.

Although regarded as very radical, interestingly enough it carries echoes of traditional medical consultation. In the good old days, the family doctor did not expect the hospital consultant to take over his patient's care. Rather, family doctor and consultant met at the domestic bedside and shared experience and specialised knowledge, with the assumption, in most cases, that both would learn from the experience and the family doctor carry on. Sometimes the consultant wouldn't tell the patient anything at all, which is sometimes quoted as a classical example of reactionary and autocratic bad manners, and perhaps it was, but the intention was that the consultant was advising the family doctor, and the family doctor was advising the patient.

This ghost of good consultation has been lost in the nonsense of imagined high technology and expertise, which is particularly inappropriate for the majority of children's emotional and behavioural problems, as shown in chapters 2 and 3. Nonetheless, social workers and psychologists, while berating the 'medical model', have failed to appreciate that the essence of the medical model is not physical diagnosis and treatment, but the concept of the expert diagnosing disorder that in theory he has the expertise to treat, and so awkward children get passed on from expert to expert and special placement when what they need is to stay in one place, with the original adults looking after them.

It is not that children should never be taken over by a more specialised group of professionals. It is simply that if the role of the child psychiatric team was clear, to themselves and to others, every referral would contain not only the possibility of the child being taken on (or in) for treatment, but also the possibility of some form of collaboration between the professionals whose help is sought, and those making the referral. Such possibilities need to be explored even when the referring agent is convinced they can do no more, because their reasons for thinking this may not be totally accurate. The request for help for a child, therefore, should be seen as an invitation to collaborate in the child's interests.

3 Questions of competence, authority and training

A recent survey of child psychiatrists in training showed how high was the interest in family therapy, and how little enthusiasm there was for prescribing drugs.[36] A debate on whether this was a good thing or not could take some time. Perhaps many children who are referred to child psychiatrists are best helped by family work, and very few by drugs. But do family therapists need to be psychiatrists? Some of the best known, and best family therapists are doctors; psychiatrists have been important innovators in the field, just as they were in psychodrama, psychoanalysis and indeed in the anti-psychiatry movement, all of which says something for the scope and qualities of medical education. But do such highly specialised therapists now really need to be trained in medicine and psychiatry first?

The point here is not that this is an urgent issue to be debated and decided, but rather that it should be a more central part of the thinking of all the professions concerned when we contemplate basic training, in-service training, the nature of new posts in the field, and the needs of troubled children. Meanwhile, if someone wants to be a competent child psychiatrist *and* a competent child psychotherapist (or family therapist) too, he or she has to ask where the time and money will come from while he or she trains and receives supervision in both.

This raises another contentious issue. First, many psychotherapists are self-taught; psychiatrists are practising what they hope or believe is psychotherapy all over the place. Who is to say whether what they are doing is 'good' or not? Committees and other bodies which try to define psychotherapy, and competent psychotherapy, or research its effectiveness soon run into major operational and conceptual difficulties. There is no one more confident, to put it politely, than the psychotherapist or family therapist who knows that his approach and personal training is the best to be had. Indeed, he may quote confidence in one's own approach as a vital ingredient in success.

A related area of disagreement is that between the collectors of data, and those who feel that the most important things in child care and child psychiatry cannot be measured. Some of these disagreements have already been referred to. If someone has the good fortune to have as colleagues people whose attitudes are at both ends of the spectrum, the valuable aspects of both can be seen. But those most competent in statistically-based academic research on the one hand, and in dealing with feelings on the other, perhaps precisely because of the meticulousness necessary to be competent in each, frequently have between them differences which are profound, and sometimes unbridgeable. Meanwhile, people muddle on in large areas of child care and treatment with only the haziest of notions about how to deal with feelings, and how to deal with data. Supervised psychotherapy and supervised research are left to the heavyweights; yet the majority of children's problems, whether seen as individual cases or in terms of an overall style of working, merit both careful object-ive appraisal *and* a more than superficial understanding of feelings.

Another source of dispute is the question of the sort of supervision needed for work with children that falls short of formal psychotherapy, yet nonetheless involves individual feelings and the relationship between worker and child. Suppose it is agreed that the person who should do important work with a child should be the person closest to the boy or girl. This may be the parents, the social worker or probation officer, or in special circumstances a residential child care worker, a nurse or perhaps a family doctor or paediatrician.

Organising supervision may be difficult for a number of reasons. First, particularly when the child is resident (for example in a special school), it may be hard to say who is doing 'key' work with the child and who isn't; one can hardly ask the child to relate only to a 'short list' of members of staff. Group supervision is possible, but there can then be problems in attendance, and the skills required to give, and benefit from, group supervision are different. Further, a 'low status' worker, charac-teristically spending most time with the child (perhaps a junior or assistant nurse or residential care worker) may not be allowed, or encouraged, to attend supervision sessions offered by a psychiatrist or psychotherapist. It may be felt by their own senior that 'work comes first', and indeed the nature of the 'low status' worker's relationship with the child may not be understood or valued. There is also the problem of the senior staff members in question feeling that they know best how to supervise their own staff, and they feel slighted by the psychiatrist or psychotherapist offering to do it instead; they may be right, or they may be wrong, but quite often it is difficult to find out, and still more difficult to make good any deficiencies, without feathers getting ruffled.

Such doubts about colleagues' competence are common. It is not just a matter of major differences in ideology, e.g. psychotherapy versus behaviour therapy. Rather, one psychotherapist may suspect another psychotherapist's approach, and not know how to raise the issue. It is even more difficult when the task is less clearly defined. A child needing particularly skilled *care*, e.g. in a children's home, may not seem to a visiting social worker to be getting it; the social worker's understanding of psychotherapy and social dynamics may feel the child's handling leaves much to be desired. But the social worker is not the care worker, and attempts to discuss misgivings can cause resentment. The social worker may also be given the message, loud and clear, that unless his or her attempts to look at the quality of handling the child is getting are carried out with extraordinary caution and tact, the staff may well feel undermined, their morale will be affected, and *then* where will we be?

Yet another problem, in a field where, as shown in chapter 5, the range of skills needed is so wide, is that of the junior member of staff who is better at some tasks than his or her senior. Some senior members of staff can cope with this better than others, and learn from the experience, but others deal with the situation by ignoring or intimidating the staff member in question, or by playing down the value of the piece of work they are doing. The problem is even greater across professions, because there is a vague hierarchy here too, with doctors generally regarded as being at the top, psychologists and social workers probably 'next equal', and nurses and residential care staff lower down. But a senior psychologist or social worker may well challenge this (or wish to), particularly when he sees a psychiatrist, for example, handling a child, family or situation less well than he would himself. And then there are the problems of trainees and juniors in each discipline: who makes decisions when there is disagreement? A middle-grade psychiatrist (say a senior registrar) or a charge nurse?

One quasi-solution is the idea of decisions by consensus, but a consensus cannot always be reached, and in any case a decision about a child cannot be determined by the relative debating skills and assertiveness of a few members of the team. Nor is the answer easily found by saying that it depends whether it is a medical or psychological or social work decision; many issues are not clearly in one or other category.

Such problems of authority, decision-making and consensus-reaching, supervision, and mutual anxieties about training and competence are potent enough difficulties when they exist among people working reasonably closely together. There is then time for people to use staff meetings and their ordinary social skills to adapt and adjust to each other and question each other's styles of work and discuss alternatives. Indeed, a team may develop excellent working relationships, each knowing the others' strengths and weaknesses and special skills and able to discuss work issues frankly and with constructive criticism. But co-operating with other people and other teams 'out there' in the community presents new difficulties; a child's problem may need people to get together who do not usually collaborate; they may not even get on with each other. A social worker or psychiatrist may refer a case for a second opinion and it may become quite clear that the local educational psychologist is just the person to help. But it then emerges that the social worker or psychiatrist has not found it possible to co-operate with the educational psychologist, or vice versa. This social work department senior, or that education welfare office, this child guidance clinic, or that adolescent unit, are 'unhelpful', 'not worth approaching', etc. Such things are very common in the field; 'it could be a first-class children's home (or school, or hostel) but we're waiting for so-and-so to retire' is heard several times a year.

4 The complexity of the subject

As shown in chapter 3, the factors that need to be taken into consideration when trying to understand children's problems are complex: many conceptually quite different facets of life interact as part of a developing and changing pattern as the child grows in his family.

To sort out the nature of children's problems, how they have developed over time, and how they interact in the present, takes collaboration between a number of different people, and takes time. Child psychiatric assessment needs time and space as basic tools. This can result in long waiting lists, which cause irritation: as mentioned in chapter 4, it may take several people several hours to do a thorough piece of work in assessing the difficulties a child and family have got into, and certainly each new family will rightly expect proper attention of this sort; but working in this way may mean that a clinic sees as many new cases in a year as, say, a surgeon might see in a couple of sessions. All the more reason, then, why child psychiatric teams should try to concentrate on children who need psychiatry; but how can they be selected as it were in advance?

Linked to this are questions of accessibility. If it is right for the child psychiatric team to try to limit the numbers of children it sees for detailed assessment and diagnosis, how can it also make itself usefully accessible for giving advice about those children the team does not see? By some means the team must obtain sufficient preliminary information, and offer sufficient genuine support and advice, to be helpful to all referring agents without seeing every child. Or should the psychiatrist or his team, as a matter of policy, see all children? And for those he does not see – for example, a child who has made suicidal threats, but whom he decides to see in a few days rather than at once – does he have substantial clinical responsibility, since he is supposed to be the expert and he has heard about the case?

5 Difficulties inherent in day-to-day work with disturbed children

Thus a practical problem is finding time to do justice to the subject. Child psychiatrists and their colleagues need to take careful histories and make detailed and thoughtful observations. One cannot find out things about worried parents and troubled children, or get to know them, by way of a hurried interrogation. Nor can decisions always be reached swiftly. Some children's cases are straightforward but the most important cases for the psychiatrist are those that are not, because parents, teachers, family doctors, social workers and others have already tried the straightforward, and perhaps some less straightforward, approaches. Decisions about whether or not time (everyone's) should be invested in regular psychotherapy or family therapy, whether or not a child should move away from home (for example into hospital, a children's home or, for the purpose of a report to a Court, into some form of care or custody) cannot be taken lightly. People who think social workers (the usual target) spend too much time in meetings and conferences often do not appreciate the difficulty and long-term consequences of the decisions that have to be reached, frequently against a background of lack of theoretical facts to go on, pressure for a firm decision, and disagreement between the various people concerned. Perhaps some of the examples quoted earlier convey the sort of dilemmas that occur. Certainly children can be found at the centre of the most complex and remarkable situations, for many of which there is no correct solution, but an arbitrary one reached by weighing up various risks, rights and demands.

The work is demanding, and many people in the field find support groups helpful or essential. Certainly time set aside for formal teaching, or learning, and for supervision, or being supervised, is essential too. As mentioned earlier, in the more hard-pressed, over-stretched circles, time for support, supervision and teaching tends to take second place to 'getting the work done', as if helping make sure that people are able to work competently is of secondary importance. The result is that the staff become even more hard-pressed and over-stretched.

On the other hand the time that could be devoted to supervision and support is unlimited: a student could spend an hour on a case, be supervised for an hour, and indeed the supervisor could spend substantial time in a senior supervisors' group too! Such things happen, particularly in orthodox psychotherapeutic circles, where it sometimes seems that nobody dares let anybody else out of their sight for a moment as far as work is concerned. There is a need for some operational studies to see how much support and supervision are needed and useful, just as there is a need for research into many of the areas mentioned in this book: which treatment helps whom? What forms of referral are most economical and helpful? What advantages are there in being taken on as a psychiatric patient, compared with receiving some other form of care? And these are comparatively coarse questions.

A lot remains to be known, not only in psychiatry, social work and psychology, but in forensic science, ethology, education, paediatrics and neurology, among many other subjects. Who is going to do this research? How are priorities going to be decided? for there is much time-wasting and paper-wasting research too. Clearly people whose main concern is clinical work, and those primarily involved in research, should collaborate closely, but this too isn't easy, and takes time.

Space as well as time is important. It may seem a mundane topic, but the fact is that many child psychiatrists and their colleagues operate in surroundings not suitable for the job. To catalogue the sorts of problems of noise, atmosphere, heating, crowding, lighting, ventilation and other basic requirements for doing the job which are frequently unmet would be tedious, but poor working conditions are common, and they are not by any means confined to adapted old buildings. It is also mentioned here, not merely in the pious hope that it may help someone, somewhere, get the waiting-room redecorated, but because such neglect is symptomatic not only of the community's ambivalent attitude to child care and child psychiatry, but because of the tendency among some child psychiatrists to belittle their own efforts, the value of their work, and the needs of their clientele.

Earlier, such mixed feelings as anxiety, uncertainty and guilt, common in the parents of troubled children, and in those involved in referral to a specialist, were mentioned. Such feelings can also arise within clinical teams. The sequence of events is fairly straightforward. Unhappy, angry children who do not readily respond to what adults do for them generate strong feelings in the adults. These strong feelings differ from adult to adult, and result in different responses; thus one adult responds to naughtiness with strictness, another with sympathy. If these were planned reactions, based on someone's theory, the situation might not be too bad, but usually the very different reactions are rooted deeply in the different adults' backgrounds, personalities and beliefs. The anxious child soon detects disagreement between those supposed to be looking after him, and becomes confused and still more anxious. He is then still harder to help, or control, at which point the adults begin overtly or covertly to blame their colleagues.

Competition about who knows best and who has the most therapeutic, 'normal' way of responding to disturbed and unhappy children is rarely far away when adults collaborate in their care, and touches on personality as well as experience. While often hidden it is more likely to become a subject for open conflict when the approach someone is taking does not seem to be working well enough, or soon enough. The position disturbed children put adults into – aroused, ambivalent, uncertain and reacting to each other closely – makes relationships between staff, as well as between staff and children, quite heated. Clinical teams working closely with children are often aware of feeling like families, albeit extended families with troubled relationships and uncomfortable relatives. Various coping devices are tried, deliberately or accidentally: staff support groups; 'sensitivity' groups; charismatic, autocratic or bureaucratic regimes; quasi-democracies, with no decisions made outside the 'community group', and so on. It is fascinating how staff relationships mirror family relationships and ultimately wider politics, with shifts of power and support, disputes about how decisions are reached and who does what, and frequent testing-out of the leadership to see how far they will go in different directions: just, democratic, authoritarian and so on, indeed whether they will stay at all, and whether they are any good, to be trusted and relied upon.

The point is not that such feelings about competition, decision-making, mutual affection and anger and the many other aspects of close collaboration in the care of children are inappropriate or pathological, to be avoided by good organisation; rather, they are inevitable, constituting the nuts and bolts of the task of co-operating and looking after children, and need to be faced and worked with. One risk is that their presence will be denied; these feelings are always present when serious work is being done in this field, and denial indicates a lack of understanding of the work, and of colleagues' feelings, that should be a cause for concern. The other risk is excessive preoccupation with such matters, so that staff become introspective and over-preoccupied with themselves instead of their work. Whatever the motives that bring people into this field, they often include feelings about childhood and parents that are still around unhelpfully in adult life, so that crises provoke individuals into behaving like little children or bossy grown-ups or whatever, and the uncomfortable feelings and memories that are provoked can lead staff to misunderstand the purpose of work done on behalf of their own feelings. This work is to help them be competent and comfortable in their job; the focus is helping with the normal difficulties of the job, and the improvement of personal skills, not therapy.

I would like to repeat the point made earlier: leaving aside for the moment the obvious importance of adult-child relationships, the bulk of the really hard and really important work done in child care and child psychiatry comes down to skilled collaboration between adults, whether we are thinking of team management, group work, running a home, school or treatment unit, investigating a child's mental retardation, finding a new school or operating a behaviour therapy programme; and it is on the nature of this collaboration that the quality of child care and child psychiatry depends. Often it founders.

Collaboration

Words in this field rapidly degenerate to jargon, reified as 'things' and even become fashionable cults. By collaboration I mean no more than working together, and in discussing this I am thinking of parents working with professionals, professionals working with each other within a team or organisation, and work between separate teams and organisations. The subject, which brings in sociology, economics, and politics as well as group dynamics, is too large to be dealt with adequately in a few pages; for the purpose of this book, I would like to do no more than remind the reader of the various ways adults work together within and between groups. I tend to use the term *liaison work* for collaboration between groups.

Why take trouble over clarifying this? Just as it was argued earlier that it was worthwhile to try to be clear about whether what one was doing was primarily treatment, training, care or control, similarly it is important to be reasonably clear about why professionals and others get together. Endless muddle and misunderstanding occur when some participants in a *decision-making meeting* think it is some sort of *support group*, and a support group can be a profound disappointment to people attending it in the hope that decisions are going to be reached.

Support
This is friendly encouragement, sharing anxieties and disappointments and affirming that the task is worthwhile and the people concerned have a chance of doing it successfully. Failing children makes adults feel like failures, and while there is not the slightest reason why adults' moods should depend on the moods of the children they are trying to look after, in fact the one is vulnerable to the other. Support reminds people of what they are able to do, and helps with the disappointment of what cannot be done.

Therapy
This is treatment, based on diagnosis and management by someone (the therapist) who purports to know more about the problem than does his client. A member of staff may well need personal help with his or her life in general, of which the day's work is part. But if so they should obtain it elsewhere. It is not the duty of colleagues to offer each other individual therapy or group therapy or marriage guidance, although if such problems emerge it is absolutely right that sympathetic advice about where to get 'extra mural' help should be available. But the help must come from outside as an individual enterprise by the member of staff, just as they might seek help for their toothache or mortgage outside.

Teaching
This refers to an aim rather than a method, because, of course, methods of teaching vary enormously. Education brings out individuals' capabilities in a given task, but also the more general skill of finding out for themselves about a task or subject. And an important part of teaching is also didactic advice and information-giving. There are times when one should help a student find out things for himself, and times when it is more sensible to explain what to do, or where to find out. *Advice-giving, information-giving*, is an important part of inter-professional liaison.

Supervision
This carries with it some responsibility for what is being done by the person being supervised. It includes elements of teaching as well as keeping an eye on progress. It is mentioned here, like teaching, because of the confusion and risk that frequently occurs when, for example, a professional thinks he is offering *consultation*, or some other form of *liaison work*, while those he is meeting with think they are being supervised. When something goes wrong this misunderstanding can stand out in sharp relief.

Consultation
This requires somewhat fuller discussion: see below.

To reiterate a point: it would be a mistake for the worker to become obsessed with the precise definition of what he is doing with his colleagues. The above modes of collaboration overlap, just as treatment and education, and care and control overlap. But it is important to acknowledge, both to oneself and sometimes in the form of an explicit if informal contract with others, what sort of work is being shared.

Consultation

'Consultation'[17,18] is used to cover a multitude of different styles of work.* The traditional medical consultation, for example, is more of an advice-giving, specialist to less-specialised, type of interaction. People say they will 'consult with' someone when they mean they will go and ask him, or go and talk things over. But consultation has been gradually acquiring its own status as a style of work, and has a special importance in child psychiatry and related fields where there is so much variation in skill, expertise, resources and in the task in hand.

In consultation, one professional helps another, on an equal basis, resolve an issue for himself. The person bringing the problem, or issue (for example, a disturbed child about whose management there is disagreement) can be called the consultee. The consultee, it is assumed, is a responsible professional with the potential for sorting the matter out for himself, but such are the uncertainties of the whole child care field that he can be helped considerably to do so if, together, consultant and consultee set up a problem-solving or issue-resolving alliance. This implies that there is skill in being a consultee, as well as being a consultant, and that is correct.

What they arrange together (and it may be one meeting about a child, a series of meetings, a group or a variety of alternative arrangements) is not to be confused with supervision or some form of therapy. It is not a teaching session (although both should learn from the experience) and it is not primarily intended for 'support', although inevitably, and appropriately, support of course emerges from a properly shared task.

* Nor should it be confused with the title *consultant*, which does not necessarily confer skill or interest in consultation as defined here.

Whether it incorporates information or advice-giving is up to the common sense of the people involved. If a social worker approaches a psychologist for help with a boy or girl for whom there is no really useful provision, and this is far from uncommon, a piece of consultative work will help the consultee decide for himself what the decisions about management will have to be, doing the best he can for the child in a far from ideal world. But if the psychologist happens to know something – perhaps a suitable residential school – the social worker clearly hasn't heard of – then this isn't kept as a secret. But there *is* a need for caution, because the consultant can be too ready to slip into advice-giving before he knows the whole story, and the consultee can fall for this before the whole story is properly explored.

What the consultee brings to the session – which may be 'one off' or a series – are:

1 His own continuing responsibility for the child, family or situation he wants to discuss. This includes the right to make up his own mind wherever he thinks the consultation has led.
2 The issue for discussion. Although the consultant's task is to help explore around the issue brought, the consultee chooses the focus.
3 His own equality, at least for the purposes of the session. This is an area of potential difficulty, and although skilled consultation does go on between people of differing status, inside or outside the same professions, if status and experience are very different there can be a 'pull' towards supervision or teaching, which the participants need to be conscious of.
4 His own resources which are:
   (a) *His own personality, training, skills, and qualities*, which it is the task of the consultant to help mobilise.
   (b) His *relationships* with the people (e.g. child or

colleague) involved with him in the subject being discussed.

(c) The *resources in his job*. This is particularly important, because it requires attention to the nature of his work and the attributes of his work setting. The tools for the job to be done are contained in, and enhanced or undermined by such things as the clarity of his role (to others as as well as himself), mutual expectations in the work he is sharing with others, time and space in which to work, agreement and clarity about the task in hand, the sort of hierarchy he works in, the opportunities for support, supervision and collaboration in general, and so on. Often the details of what makes a job possible, or undermines it, occupy as blind a spot as does unconscious motivation.

Consultation in child psychiatry: some conclusions

The task of consultation – which is where the consultant's skill comes in – is to set the scene for the *nature of the problem and the needs of the child or situation to be adequately explored and clarified as a joint enterprise*. This may be relatively brief – perhaps over the phone – or it may require a separate and prolonged meeting, perhaps more than one. Thus two professionals experienced at consultation should be able to agree, on the basis of a two or three minute 'phone call, whether, for example, the situation is one that requires an immediate decision, whatever the risks; or that an immediate decision is inappropriate, but that a longer consultation is going to be needed, e.g. tomorrow or next week.

A central place for consultation as a skill in child care and child psychiatry does *not* mean that professional workers would be endlessly chewing things over together, instead of dashing about making decisions and giving 'therapy'. If the point of consultation was clear and agreed, collaboration would be increasingly brisk and efficient, because it would become clearer where the most time needed to be spent and where the deficiencies were, which is child psychiatry's greatest need, in overall planning as well as in the case of the individual child or family.

With anxiety, muddle and evasion formally dealt with, it might become crystal clear that what is needed is, to take a few examples: a different support structure in a children's home; a detailed diagnostic appraisal of a child who does indeed seem to have something 'wrong' within; a change of school, or a change of approach by teaching staff; better teaching and supervision in a particular area of work; an aspect of functioning or method about which everyone is ignorant and which needs researching; that a child cannot be coped with by any of the means available, and for everyone's sake must be securely contained; that a firmer line must be taken with a junior, a senior or other colleague; or that the consultee has found *for himself* a gap in his training or an aspect of his personality or attitudes that is making the job difficult, and that he must decide for himself what to do about it. Role-examination may even reveal that a particular role is redundant.

It is not that consultation never happens. It goes on here and there, sometimes, more or less. But the nature of child psychiatry and its use by other professions and by the community in general, its expense, the time it takes to do properly and the fact that so many children need something *other than* child psychiatry or something *as well* as child psychiatry, means that a) consultation within and across the specialties should be far more skilled and helpful than it is at present, and b) clarifying who wants or needs what, and who is in the best position to provide it, is fundamental and essential at every level – individual and in terms of planning and organisation.

A consultative approach to each problem surrounding a child, as it arises, would help clarify matters; but as can be seen from the brief examples given, what emerges may be surprising, and acting on it will sometimes take effort and courage.

8

The Uses of Child Psychiatry: Conclusions

Nothing is more important than the proper care and education of children. If this is good enough, everything else follows. The part to be played by child psychiatry and its allied disciplines, however, in contributing to the care and education of children risks being over-emphasised. This is not only because its approach in individual cases is not always helpful, but because the very principle of a growing (and already large) band of highly trained, high status professional workers with supposedly extra special technical expertise in the understanding and management of troubled children (whose numbers grow ever greater as more problems are defined) may undermine parents and teachers more than it helps them. In a book that is largely forgotten (although not by George Orwell[69] when the ideas that led to *1984* were taking shape), Burnham proposed that the greatest threat to freedom was not from capitalism nor socialism, but from a growing army of managers, bureaucrats, organisers and technical experts, well-meaning democratic liberals all.

There is no easy answer to this. I agree with Rutter and Madge[86] when they say that many of the problems of disadvantaged children will not be changed by massive social and economic changes in our social structure, and those with experience of children's problems know how many are clearly rooted in the facts of biological and emotional life and growth and not in terms of social factors alone. *And yet* if experts (child psychiatrists, educational psychologists, family therapists *et al*) are needed to help parents and teachers with 20, 30 or 40 per cent of the children in some areas (and it is not difficult to make a case for such levels of 'disorder') does this not challenge the very idea of what is *normal*, which ought to be in the province of ordinary people, teachers, writers, poets, and legislators, rather than left to technical experts in abnormality? If one child in five is likely to need special education at some point in his school career, as the Warnock Committee reported,[26] then we need to reconsider what is properly within the province of normal education; fortunately current thinking is that special education does not have to be in 'special' centres. A similar philosophical muddle occurs in considering delinquency. There is a major gap between individually-orientated criminologists who can say with some accuracy that *these children in these circumstances behave this way*, and develop their thinking from there, and the more socially and culturally orientated who say that a community will generate various forms of dissent and deviation and rule-breaking, and that should be the perspective, not the individual case.

There is no doubt that many expert (and expensively achieved) observations and methods of intervention are valuable and effective. The question mark is over how such knowledge should be used, a point to be referred to later.

Common sense versus complexity

Common sense is neither good nor bad; it is just what most people happen to believe. A community or culture agreed on its own needs will learn through its teachers and philosophers, using these terms in their widest sense, how to cope with problems outside the capacity of general common sense and skill. In earlier times, the message from, say, physician or clergyman was as often to put up with the problem, or get rid of the awkward child or person, as it was advice on how to help, e.g. with special prayers or potions. It is the special help that has now expanded into a vast, rich and burgeoning general scientific technology that might do absolutely anything for any problem, given the time and money.

If common sense – that which is commonly believed, and commonly effective – about caring for, disciplining and educating children fails to work, uncommon sense is called for. Supposing competent and responsible parents and skilled teachers have tried all they know with a child in difficulties, and in many cases they will know a great deal, the child may be referred to a child psychiatric team. As discussed earlier in the book, there are two broad aspects to this request and two general responses:

1 Helping the parents and teachers cope, with the additional support, advice and information they need.
2 Recognising that this child does indeed have an individual problem that requires help that it is unreasonable to expect parents and teachers to give.

The first area of work is educative and consultative, and takes into account the fact that parents and teachers, closest to the child, in more contact with him, and in a normal as opposed to artificial setting, should be able to do the necessary work better than professionals, as in the recent developments in helping autistic and mentally handicapped children via their parents.

The second area of work is the more traditional treatment of the individual boy or girl by a specialist trained, and with the time as well as the expertise, to carry out a treatment programme. But it can also include special care, control and education which in the same way is more demanding, and more time-consuming than common sense methods can cope with.

Where the psychotherapies, various counselling methods and family therapy fit in with these alternatives is controversial. Counselling at its best, between professional and client, is like consultation between professional and professional: the consultant (or counsellor) makes no diagnosis, but enables the consultee (or person being counselled) to make up his own mind about how best to use his own resources. Counselling and consultation would therefore go into the first category, with advice and information-giving. What they all have in common is a broadly *educative* approach, not diagnosing the individual but helping him do his best and be able to operate more independently and imaginatively in future.

Many forms of psychotherapy and family therapy are like this, aiming at personal (or family) development, rather than curing disorder. But undoubtedly many psychotherapists (though they may deny it) unconsciously work as though the individual or the family were sick. Some psychotherapy and family therapy comes into the first category, and some into the second, depending on the therapist's ideology and style.

The referral sequence: common sense to complexity

What is being suggested is an ideal sequence for dealing with children who are in difficulties.

The three stages are:

1 Education

One of the most important responsibilities of those with special understanding and skills is to feed them back to everyone else. This may happen in the case of the individual child (e.g. reassurance that a particular

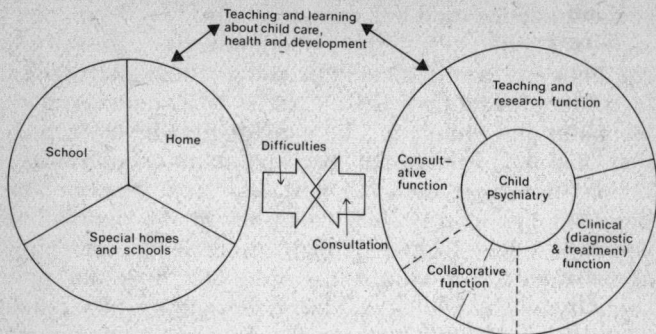

Fig. 7 A conceptual model for a child and adolescent psychiatry service.

Aims

1 Prevention (via learning and teaching and work-focused consultation).

2 When problems arise, emphasis on helping the adults already involved to continue using their own resources: i.e. consultative work.

3 If this is insufficient, some technical and advisory assistance from child psychiatric team: i.e. collaborative work.

   For a minority of children presenting emotional and behavioural problems taking them on for treatment.

pattern of behaviour is part of normal development) or it may be part of the general process by which new knowledge is gradually disseminated. Health education is not always informed or skilled, and very often the already best informed groups tend to go for more; good education by schools, perhaps involving parents, with a gradual filtering into the community of what the experts are uncovering, with pros and cons presented too, is perhaps better than massive and dogmatic propaganda campaigns.

2   Consultation

This refers not only to consultation about a child with an identified problem, but *consultation about the referral*. The more it could be accepted on both sides that the contribution of child psychiatry to the particular child's case is *usually* in doubt, that the people already involved can *usually* do more than they may realise, and that this, and the possibilities of collaboration, deserve to be explored, the more likely it will be that very specialised resources (with their cost in money, time and side-effects) can be kept for the very small minority who need them.

The distinction between consultation and counselling needs explanation. The difference is more of aim rather than process. In *consultation*, which is with a 'front line' professional already called in (e.g. family doctor, clergyman, social worker), the discussion is job-focused. In *counselling*, with someone in a non-professional parenting position, the focus is inevitably somewhat more personal, concerned with individual hopes, aspirations and caring rather than professional relationships, for example with the child, other children and husband or wife.

3   Diagnosis and treatment

This will always consider aspects of care, education and discipline whether treatment as such is needed or not, and follows if consultation reveals that there is a useful place for this approach. But note that complex diagnosis does not necessarily result in complex solutions. Clarification may be hard work but result in simpler strategies which help than was thought possible.

Two points need to be made about this sequence. First, a series of barriers to treatment, making the child psychiatrist and his colleagues less accessible is *not* being proposed. Rather, I am suggesting that a most important part of the child psychiatric team's repertoire should be its educational and consultative function, teaching, advising, reassuring where reassurance is appropriate, directing to other sources of help when necessary, and consulting, with the move to the diagnostic and treatment process being held very much in reserve. Perhaps a good analogy would be with the ideal family doctor who would refer to hospital rarely, prescribe drugs infrequently, offer advice, support and perhaps counselling (*not* psychotherapy) often. He would still recognise the major disease that occasionally came his way, and arrange what was needed within minutes, hours or days, but his skill would also be in recognising when such action was not needed.

This leads to the second point, and which was referred to in an earlier chapter. What is being proposed is not lots of talk to put off action. Usually more usefully directed discussion is indeed needed, but if there was far more awareness of the differing needs of different children, and hazy and misleading concepts of 'disturbance' and 'psychotherapy' out of the way, a helpfully and skilfully collaborating adult world, parent, teacher and specialist would far more easily be able to agree when a swift decision was needed, for example that a child's neglect or behaviour was intolerable and must be brought to a stop *now* (not 'perhaps', after a six-week wait for the child psychiatrist's report), or that a boy or girl was quite clearly psychiatrically ill and should be in hospital today.

And if such things were clarified, the adult world could deal more confidently with the wild and destructive (and self-destructive) behaviour that young children get away with for *years*, to their own cost, while people wonder whether they need birching or psychoanalysis; and children whose need is for extra order and caring in their lives would not accumulate in psychiatric units for young people.

Proper consultation would lead to the right decisions and, eventually, the setting up of the right resources. But useful consultation will not take place until more professionals appreciate that it takes considerable skill to consult, as well as to be consulted. Nor will the right resources stand a chance of emerging until what is missing, and what is needed, are clarified and agreed, which is as much a task for consultation as for research.

Diagnosis, treatment and the multi-professional team

The problem not resolved by information, advice or consultation alone will therefore need a different sort of appraisal: since common sense and ordinary measures have failed, even when extra advice and support has been tried, and consultation has enabled the exploring of all possible alternatives, then the problem needs examination along less straightforward and simple lines. *Uncommon* sense is needed: the special knowledge and language of psychodynamic theory, or neuro-development, or family systems theory, or biochemistry. Moreover, the special skill of putting such things together in a way that make sense, as described in chapters 3 and 4.

The very fact that a wide range of skills is needed to do this, and to institute the management the diagnosis points to, raises a new problem. Two, three or more people with considerable experience in quite different yet overlapping fields are needed, and this very difference, and the overlap, makes collaboration potentially difficult.

The personality and training needed to be good at identifying abnormalities in a child's behaviour or mental state are not the same as those needed to be a good family therapist or social worker. The various sorts of psychologist (the careful measures, behaviour therapists and psychotherapists) are different again. Their beliefs, views of the world and politics – certainly their salaries – will be different. And they will usually have strong feelings and views about the definition of abnormality, the diagnostic process, methods of treatment, and about how the team should be organised, and who should be in charge and set the style of work. They are likely to be quite individualistic people, with strong motives, for good or ill, that have brought them into this kind of work.

Not only will their professional backgrounds and the journals they read be different, they will have different allegiances, and very often they will be operating from quite different professional hierarchies. A child psychiatric (or child guidance) clinic is likely to be run by a Health Authority, Education Department and Social Services Department in more or less uncomfortable liaison. Sometimes it works well, but the unhappy conflict and intrigue that also goes on can be beyond belief: different departments battling for the 'control' of the child psychiatrist (when appointed), or arguing over who should pay for the curtains, since in Department A's arrangements they are part of the fabric of the building but Department B regards them as furniture. These and other distractions can occupy the clinical team for years, and to an extent that would astonish people who want help for their children.

A hospital department can have similar problems, with medical, nursing, social work, teaching and other hierarchies tussling for their views to prevail, their needs to be met, their ambitions to be fulfilled. These and other problems were elaborated in chapter 7, and the point made that nonetheless the nature of children's problems requires the adults to work sensibly together and make decisions in uncertain, unpredictable and sometimes very risky situations with relatively little in the way of firm guidelines.

The role of the child psychiatrist

Many of the problems described through this book are unavoidable, being inherent in the nature of the disorder, the various forms of response, and the overlap between the professionals who have to work together. But although it would be impossible on theoretical grounds and in the interests of day-to-day practice to demarcate rigidly the different professional roles, the *focus* of each role should be clear.

Other professions should define their own role; I would like to do this for child and adolescent psychiatry, and this may help others define their own function. Medical registration alone permits the prescription of dangerous drugs and the signing of certain statutory certificates, but little else. What is there about the child psychiatrist's training that qualifies him for the work that has been described?

1   The nature of the medical model

As argued earlier in the book and elsewhere,[106] the special nature of the much maligned medical model is not a preference for physical causes and treatment, but the diagnosis of individual abnormality. A key role of the child psychiatrist is the identification of individual disorder – whether psychodynamic or biological or a combination of these in the individual child. The ability to think in terms of a number of quite different levels of function, as described in chapters 3 and 4, is a further component of the medical attitude. Doctors may not be invariably expert in thinking in psychological, social, neurological, biochemical and other terms in whatever combination seems to be nearest to an accurate description of the problem, but their training makes this possible, and provides a basis for further professional development along these lines. It is fashionable to criticise doctors; and their training, with its emphasis on, say, detailed anatomy and surgical technique, and the lack of skill many doctors have in dealing with people's feelings when they qualify, certainly don't make them automatically suited for psychiatric training. And yet, if a course were to be devised to train people for the task of a child psychiatrist as defined here, it would be nearer to medical training than anything else, and at least as long too, with perhaps more emphasis on anthropology, general biology, psychology, sociology and training in interview and consultative techniques; but still a recognisable medical course.

Moreover, medical training is not inflexible, and by the time a medical student has become a child psychiatrist he or she will often have gained experience, within formal training and outside, in the more appropriate medical-social-psychological fields. It is easy to criticise doctors, and some of the most vehement criticism of doctors who have spent ten to fifteen years or more in such training come from those with only three years undergraduate study of, say, sociology, psychology or politics.

The doctor is therefore well equipped to be an explorer of new fields, of which ethology[46, 49] is an important example, which is useful as the direction psychiatry in particular ought to take is uncertain. Certainly by nature and status doctors can be stick-in-the-mud in character, but equally, as mentioned in an earlier chapter, doctors have pioneered such variegated fields as psychodrama, gestalt therapy, psychoanalysis, family therapy, the therapeutic community and even 'anti-psychiatry'.

2 Psychiatric skills

These include at their core the assessment of the individual's mental state, the gradually acquired ability to understand from posture, word or gesture whether someone is a little unhappy or suicidally, perhaps homicidally, depressed; a little sensitive or in a paranoid state; muddled or thought disordered; excited or manic. Children's mental states differ from those of adults, but the principle and discipline is similar, and the assessment and treatment of the mental state of older members of the family is an important part of child psychiatry too.

3 General medical skills

These are not striking in psychiatrists but by and large they know when they are out of their depth, they use the language of other sorts of doctor, they tend to be able to recognise the signs of ill health even if they may need to consult with others about detailed diagnosis, and they know enough to treat children with, say, anorexia nervosa, cut wrists, belly-aches, incontinence, head-aches, 'dizzyness', 'feeling sick', epilepsy and acne without constant reference to other doctors. Withdrawn, depressive and schizophrenic states can be alarming, and puzzle general physicians too, and psychiatrists are usually able to monitor general nutrition and levels of consciousness while keeping the young person (who may also be on drugs) under psychiatric supervision, managing much better than when a psychiatrically disturbed child or adolescent is on a general medical ward. On a more general note, the relationship with general medicine, paediatrics and neurology is two-way, and these specialties gain from close professional contact with psychiatry as well as vice versa.

4 Drugs

The use of drugs and monitoring their effects and side effects is an important part of child psychiatry, or should be: see page 115.

5 Monitoring the effects of any treatment

This occurs once a multi-dimensional formulation of problems has been made, and is, after all, a matter of repeating diagnosis in order to check progress.

6 Having the authority to say that there is no psychiatric disorder

This is too little used by some psychiatrists.

7 Co-ordination

Being able to co-ordinate the work of people who can work in the technical areas referred to, in the interests of the child, who may be having, for example, medication, family therapy, special teaching and nursing.

Having listed the special contribution the psychiatrist can make to a team dealing with difficult-to-understand children, it is necessary to add what can be done without needing a psychiatric background. It is not necessary to be a psychiatrist to do or teach psychotherapy, family therapy, consultation, to run a therapeutic community or a service or residential setting designed for special care, control or special education. And, if the argument of this book has been followed, it will be clear that the case for more skills and resources in these areas is perhaps on firmer foundations than the case for 'more psychiatry'.

Leadership of the multi-professional team

This is a hot issue at the moment, with much fighting (hand-to-hand, as well as between the general staff) over who should be in charge of child guidance and child psychiatric clinics, although there are attempts to blur the issue with fashionable euphemisms such as 'co-ordination' and 'facilitation' rather than leadership. A professional team dealing with disturbed children and their families requires definite leadership, which is not the same as saying autocratic or authoritarian leadership; it must be a leadership which respects the professional roles of others in the team. If the core function of the team is *psychiatric*, leadership should come from a psychiatrist. If it is primarily psychotherapeutic, or geared to family therapy, or caring, controlling or educative, then the job should go to the most appropriately experienced and qualified. Presumably psychiatrists, suitably trained, would not be excluded from applying.

Dealing with the difficulties inherent in the work

These difficulties were described in chapter 7 and will not be repeated here.

1   The special problems and needs of working with disturbed children must be emphasised forcefully and repeatedly to organisers and administrators who may be admirable people but who are often woefully ignorant of the demands of working with difficult children, in psychiatry or outside. The way in which children's homes and psychiatric units are staffed by residential care workers and nurses respectively is often scandalous, with over-stretched, unsupported, undertrained and inadequately supervised people, often young and inexperienced, moving rapidly from job to job.

2   Innovation and experiment, if sensibly planned, should be encouraged. In particular, shared training between people in different parts of the field, work outside residential units (e.g. day unit, domiciliary and out-patient work, fostering, consultation with other teams and units) should be encouraged to open up work that is going on in isolated compartments. Formal research, which needs training, is essential, but so is the fostering of a spirit of imaginative enquiry about what we are doing and, if it helps, time for study, discussion and research projects should be built into the work; there is too much ignorance around for this to be a luxury or an optional extra.

3   Workers in this field need a considerable measure of autonomy. Children and parents in trouble need the authoritative and personal advice of the professional worker as an individual, not the 'department view'. Doctors have, so far, managed to keep a considerable degree of professional autonomy once in a fully

trained position (as consultant) but social workers and nurses are rapidly losing themselves in complex bureaucratic hierarchies and should do what they can as professions to counteract this trend. Teams and units too, should as far as possible be responsible for their own work with their own patients and clients, and with the boss on the premises.

4 As with supervision and teaching built inextricably into the job, there is a need for training and skill in consultation. All that has been said about consultation between the referring professional worker and the specialist team applies also to working relationships between members of the team. The difficulties in the field are an integral part of it, and will never go away; anyone training in child psychiatry and related fields should be experienced in the sort of skills needed for collaborating and consulting with other professions in their own team and outside. This requires training. The 'multi-disciplinary team' which held out such high hopes sixty years ago has still not generated much in the way of serious thought about how such teams should work effectively and imaginatively, nor indeed why many have failed to do so.

5 The function of the team, service or unit, and the role of its members of staff, should be as clear as possible. Sometimes total clarity in this developing, dynamic, and ambiguous field would result in undue rigidity. Nonetheless, just as the team should assume and anticipate inter-worker problems and have ways of coping with them, similarly there should be a consciousnes and expectation that from time to time roles and goals should be clarified and reaffirmed as far as possible. What is needed is not a neatly tied-up solution to all these problems, but constant maintenance.

Conclusions

Child and adolescent psychiatry should re-examine its role and redefine it more closely, which means that it should limit its clientele. This means that it should reduce the number of children regarded as psychiatrically disturbed in the community. This is because we know that many of the children who come the way of psychiatrists, and some of whom are helped by them, do not actually need psychiatry.

We should also be more cost-conscious. Child psychiatry is an expensive exercise, and should limit its expertise in diagnosis and treatment to the limited number of children who are shown by educative and consultative approaches as needing more meticulous, biological, social and psychological assessment. But this means better educational, consultative and collaborative work with non-psychiatric services, as well as the highest standard of diagnosis and treatment for the children who do 'filter through' to psychiatry. Whether this means we will ultimately need more child psychiatrists or less is hard to say without reference to local conditions; many areas at home and in developing countries may need more, but even then the sort of child psychiatrists needed will be those who can enable a broad-based service to evolve in which other professions (preferably not too profligate in number) can do the work for which medical training isn't needed.

One consequence of this deliberately more limited role should be that its academic aspects, both research and teaching, again in collaboration with those outside psychiatry, should be developed as its treatment role is more tightly restricted to those who really need it. It should confine its clinical practice and study to the most intractable problems such as those needing multi-dimensional assessment and treatment, helping others do more straightforward work. It should become an ex-perimental, exploratory, teaching subject, with serious mental illness as its main clinical concern. And research does not invariably have to be an elaborate, costly exercise; an exploratory, innovatory, imaginative style of work, able to tolerate and assess new ideas and consider both minor shifts of emphasis and radical changes of direction, should be part of the repertoire of all specialties within the child care and treatment field. Consultation, as described earlier, is one of the tools of this form of trade. Inquiry should focus on *prevention* of problems, their *early identification* and clarifying which responses are most helpful. These are still largely open questions.

Another consequence of this deliberately more limited role would be the encouragement of other professions and services to define their own roles, and develop in their own way, taking part in collaborative planning to avoid duplication of function, and gaps in services, research and training. At present, not only do we have gaps, we have too many super-specialists pressing for a role in each child's case, convinced that certain work cannot proceed without their own involvement. We need to learn more from each other, and then the number of individual professionals working with each child and family could be far less. This step will require better and wider individual professional training, which will then allow more mutual trust between professional workers, so that one or two people will be allowed to get on with the job without endless checking and reviewing and 'communicating'; but unfortunately, the way people are trained and supervised at present does work against the development of reasonably autonomous 'general practitioners' in child treatment and care.

The child psychiatric team would make itself more accessible, not less, offering information, advice and consultation while also maintaining the aim of taking on for diagnosis and treatment fewer children than is the case at present. But it would not do this responsibly without actively working for the right services and professionals being available, trained and supported, outside psychiatry; a well staffed, properly supported children's home, for example, rather than another in-patient unit.

In some areas child psychiatry might have to expand a little; for example in the rather unpopular area of looking after the small but accumulative number of children with chronic psychotic disorders who need nursing and medical care and cannot be looked after by child care workers or teachers alone.

At all costs we must encourage more continuity of care, over several years in the cases of some children and families, and all professions must look carefully at ways in which their career structures operate directly against providing the very stability and constancy of professional relationships at the core of many children's needs.

In suggesting this gentle but insistent 'pushing back' of as many problems as possible and practicable to parents, teachers, and caring and controlling resources, always with help, I am not suggesting a sudden change of direction, but a developing shift of emphasis, with the wider community being helped to see that it can do more than it thinks for children without psychiatric intervention; or, where psychiatry is helpful, that it makes a contribution rather than takes over completely. Ideally, the other specialised professions would take a similar approach. How can specialist professions and academic centres helpfully inform the general public about normal child care and development (as once they educated the community in the basic rules of public health) without putting people at the mercy of a stream of idiosyncratic and conflicting 'correct views' flowing from this or that Institute or Department or pressure group? Experience so far is far from reassuring.

This might seem a lot to ask of child psychiatrists: a gradual giving up of the more readily soluble problems, or those that really do not need multi-factorial assessment and management, back to simpler, more direct and perhaps less expensive systems of care, education and control. Areas of work would be given up to psychotherapists, psychologists, social workers and teachers because the child's and family's needs were more clearly in their areas of expertise, whether 'easier' or not. Psychiatry for children would return towards its roots, trying to fathom the un-understandable, as did its earlier practitioners, who were called *alienists*. So much that what was once non-understandable is now understandable, in terms of psychodynamics, behavioural psychology, family and social dynamics, and having taken part in exploring these areas of understanding, and developing other methods and other professions, child psychiatry should think about its withdrawal.

The specialty would have to change substantially to achieve this, with a redistribution of interests, skills and resources; although a redefinition of its role, with the encouragement of others concerned with children to redefine theirs, would make all forms of collaboration more fruitful, not less. Perhaps this change could be seen as growth, with gains as well as losses, and as a necessary next stage in the maturation of the specialty.

Recommended Reading

1   Short accounts of child and adolescent psychiatry and development

Short books need to be read even more critically than large ones, because inevitably there is less room for the author to discuss conflicting opinions, even if he or she wanted to. The following are good, fairly brief accounts of the approaches of some prominent practitioners.

Basic Child Psychiatry, J C Barker, London: Crosby Lockwood Staples, 1979.

The Nature of Adolescence, J C Coleman, London: Methuen and Co., 1980.

Growing Pains, E M Irwin, Plymouth: Macdonald and Evans, 1977.

Helping Troubled Children, M Rutter, Harmondsworth: Penguin Books, 1972.

Maternal Deprivation Reassessed, M Rutter, Harmondsworth: Penguin Books, 1972.

Children Under Stress, S Wolff, Harmondsworth: Penguin Books, 1974.

Changing Youth in a Changing Society, M Rutter, London, The Nuffield Provincial Hospitals Trust. Good, comprehensive account of adolescent development and epidemiology.

2   For reference

Child Psychiatry: Modern Approaches, ed M Rutter and L Hersov, Oxford, Blackwell Scientific Publications, 1977. A

large, comprehensive book and a good source of references.
Education, Health and Behaviour, M Rutter, J Tizard and
K Whitmore, London: Longman, 1970. An important
epidemiological study of children's difficulties in a particular population (the Isle of Wight).

3   Psychodynamic theory and therapy

The literature is too large and variegated to provide a really
useful short list. The text of this book and the list of
references shows some of the author's own preferences; I have
found the work of Anna Freud,[33] Melanie Klein,[53] John
Bowlby,[8,9,10,11] Erik Erikson[19,30] and Donald Winnicott[112,113]
particularly helpful. For family theory, see e.g. Christopher
Dare[24,74] and Robin Skynner.[95] J A C Brown's small book on
Freudian theory[12] and its developments is one of the best
introductions to psychoanalytic theory. Wyss's book[118] is
excellent for more detail.

Do not neglect the many examples of observations on
children to be found in classical and modern literature.

4   Journals

For developments in child and adolescent psychiatry and
related disciplines it is worth keeping an eye on the *Journal of
Child Psychology and Psychiatry* (Pergamon Press), which is
the journal of the Association for Child Psychology and
Psychiatry, and the *Journal of Adolescence* (Academic Press)
which is the journal of the Association for the Psychiatric
Study of Adolescence. Both organisations are multidisciplin-
ary, and despite their titles have a very heterogenous member-
ship. The former is the more academically-orientated of the
two.

References

1 Barker, P *The Residential Psychiatric Treatment of Children*, London, Crosby Lockwood Staples, 1974.
2 —— *Basic Child Psychiatry*, London, Crosby Lockwood Staples, 1979.
3 Berger, M, Howlin, P, Marchant, R, Hersov, L, Rutter, M and Yule, W 'Instructing Parents in the Use of Behaviour Modification Techniques as Part of a Home-based Approach to the Treatment of Autistic Children', *Behaviour Modification Newsletter*, 5, 15–27, 1973.
4 Berkowitz, B P and Graziano, A M 'Training Parents as Behaviour Therapists: A Review,' *Behaviour Research and Therapy*, 10, 297–317, 1972.
5 Brewer, C and Lait, J *Can social work survive?* London, Temple-Smith, 1980.
6 Blos, P 'The Second Individuation Process of Adolescence', *Psychoanal. Study of the Child*, 22, 162–186, 1967.
7 Blumberg, H 'Drug taking', in 85, 1977.
8 Bowlby, J 'Attachment and Loss', Vol. 1, *Attachment*, Harmondsworth, Penguin.
9 —— 'Attachment and Loss', Vol. 2, *Separation: Anxiety and Anger, Ibid*, 1973.
10 —— 'Attachment and Loss', Vol. 3, *Loss*, London, Hogarth, 1979.
11 —— *The Making and Breaking of Affectional Bonds*, London, Tavistock, 1979.
12 Brown, J A C *Freud and the post-Freudians*, Harmondsworth, Penguin, 1961.

13 Bruggen, P, Byng-Hall, J and Pitt-Aikens, T 'The reason for admission as a focus of work for an adolescent unit', *Brit. J. Psychiat.*, 122, 319–329, 1973.

14 Bruggen, P and Westland, P 'Difficult to Place Adolescents: Are More Resources Required?' *Journal of Adolescence*, 2, 245–250, 1979.

15 Cadbury, G S *Young Offenders Yesterday and Today*, London, George Allen and Unwin, 1938.

16 Cantwell, D 'Hyperkinetic syndrome', in 85, 1977.

17 Caplan, G *Principles of Preventive Psychiatry*, London, Tavistock, 1964.

18 —— The Theory and Practice of Mental Health Consultation, London, Tavistock, 1970.

19 Chisholm, D D 'Obesity in adolescence', *Journal of Adolescence*, 1, 177–194, 1978.

20 Connell, P 'Clinical aspects of drug misuse', in 85, 1977.

21 Corbett, J 'Tics and Tourette's Syndrome', in 85, 1977.

22 Crisp, A H, Palmer, R L and Kalucy, R S 'How common is anorexia nervosa? A prevalence study', *Brit. J. Psychiat.* 128, 549–554, 1976.

23 Crisp, A H *Anorexia nervosa*, London, Academic Press, 1980.

24 Dare, C 'A Classification of Interventions in Child and Conjoint Family Therapy', *Psychotherapy and Psychosomatics*, 25, 116–125, 1975.

25 Department of Health and Social Security, 'Fit for the future', Report of the Committee on Child Health Services, S D M Court, London, HMSO, 1976.

26 Department of Education and Science, 'Special educational needs', Report of the Committee of Enquiry into the Education of Handicapped Children and Young People, H M Warnock, London, HMSO, 1978.

27 De Mause, L (Ed), *The History of Childhood*, London, Souvenir Press Ltd, 1974.

28 Eisenberg, L 'The Ethics of Intervention: Acting Amidst Ambiguity', *J. Child Psychology and Psychiatry*, 16, 93–104, 1975.

29 Erikson, E H *Childhood and Society*, Harmondsworth, Penguin, 1967.

30 Erikson, E H *Identity: Youth and Crisis*, London, Faber and Faber, 1968.

31 Flexner, A 'Is social work a profession?', Proceedings of the National Conference of Charities and Corrections, 1915.

32 Foucault, M *Madness and Civilisation*, London, Tavistock, 1967.

33 Freud, A *Normality and Pathology in Childhood*, Harmondsworth, Penguin, 1973.

34 Freud, S *Introductory Lectures on Psychoanalysis*, London, George Allen and Unwin, 1922.

35 Freudenberger, H J 'The Staff Burnout Syndrome in Alternative Institutions', *Psychotherapy*, Spring 1975, 73–82, 1975.

36 Garralda, M E, 'Trainees' attitudes in child psychiatry', *Bulletin of the Royal College of Psychiatrists*, 26–7, February 1980.

37 Graham, P and Rutter, M 'Psychiatric Disorder in the Young Adolescent – a Follow-up Study', *Proceedings of the Royal Society of Medicine*, 66, 1226–9, 1973.

38 Green, R 'Atypical psychosexual development,' in 85, 1977.

39 Harris, R 'The EEG (Electroencephalogram)', in 85, 1977.

40 Hazel, N 'Family Placement – a Hopeful Alternative', *Journal of Adolescence*, 1, 363–9, 1978.

41 Hersov, L A 'Emotional Disorders', in 85, 1977.

42 —— 'Faecal Soiling', in 85, 1977.

43 —— 'School Refusal', in 85, 1977.

44 Hersov, L A, Berger, M and Nicol, A R (Eds), *Language and Language Disorders*, Pergamon, Oxford, 1980.

45 Hibbert, C, *The Roots of Evil. A Social History of Crime and Punishment*, London, Weidenfeld and Nicolson, 1963.

46 Hinde, R A 'On describing relationships', *Journal of Child Psychology and Psychiatry*, 17, 1–19, 1976.

47 Hoghughi, M *Troubled and Troublesome. Coping with Severely Disordered Children*, London, André Deutsch, 1978.

48 Humphrey, G *The Wild Boy of Aveyron*, New York, The Century Company, 1932.

49 Hutt, S J 'The role of behaviour studies in psychiatry: an ethological viewpoint', *Behaviour Studies in Psychiatry*, S J Hutt and C Hutt (Eds), Oxford, Pergamon, 1970.

50   Johnson, C A and Katz, R C 'Using Parents as Change
       Agents for their Children: A Review', *Journal of Child
       Psychology and Psychiatry*, 14, 181–200, 1973.

51   Jones, M *Social Psychiatry in Practice: The Idea of a
       Therapeutic Community*, Harmondsworth, Penguin,
       1968.

52   Kalucy, R S 'An Approach to the Therapy of Anorexia
       Nervosa', *Journal of Adolescence*, 1, 197–228, 1978.

53   Klein, M *Envy and gratitude*, London, Tavistock, 1957.

54   Kreitman, N *Parasuicide*, Chichester, Wiley, 1977.

55   Laing R D *The Divided Self*, Harmondsworth, Penguin,
       1965.

56   Leach, E Fifth Aubrey Lewis Lecture, given at the
       Institute of Psychiatry, 9 November, 1977.

57   Leslie, S A 'Psychiatric Disorder in the Young Ado-
       lescents of an Industrial Town', *Brit. J. Psychiat.*, 125,
       113–24, 1974.

58   Lewis, A 'Social aspects of psychiatry', *Edinburgh
       Medical Journal*, 58, 241–7, 1951.

59   Lubove, R *The Professional Altruist: The Emergence of
       Social Work as a Career 1880–1930*, Cambridge,
       Massachusetts, Harvard University Press, 1971.

60   Lynch, M, Steinberg, D and Ounsted, C 'A family unit
       in a children's psychiatric hospital', *Brit. Med. J.* 2,
       127–129, 1975.

61   Maslach, C 'Burned-out', *Human Behaviour*, 5, 16–22,
       1976.

62   Masterton, G 'The management of Solvent Abuse',
       Journal of Adolescence, 2, 65–75, 1979.

63   Menzies, I *The Functioning of Social Systems as a
       Defence Against Anxiety*, London, Tavistock Institute
       of Human Relations, 1970.

64   —— 'Staff Support Systems. Task and Anti-task in
       Adolescent Institutions', *Proceedings of the Ninth
       Annual Conference of the Association for the Psy-
       chiatric Study of Adolescence*, 1974.

65   Meyer, V and Chesser, E S *Behaviour Therapy in
       Clinical Psychiatry*, Harmondsworth, Penguin, 1970.

66   Milham, S, Bullock, R and Hosie, K *Locking up
       Children: Secure Provision Within the Child Care
       System*, Farnborough, Hants, Saxon Press, 1978.

67   Newsome, A 'Doctors and counsellors: collaboration or

conflict?' *Bulletin of the Royal College of Psychiatrists*, 102–104, July 1980.

68 Newsome, A, Thorne, B J and Wyld K L *Student Counselling in Practice*, London, University of London Press, 1975.

69 Orwell, G 'James Burnham and the Managerial Revolution' (1942, Putnam, London), in *Collected Essays, Journalism and Letters of George Orwell*, 1946. (Eds. S Orwell and I Angus) Harmondsworth, Penguin, 1970.

70 Penrose, L S *Mental Defect*, London, Sidgwick and Jackson, 1933.

71 Piaget *The Language and Thought of the Child*, London, Kegan Paul, Trench and Trubner, 1926.

72 —— *The Origins of Intelligence in the Child*, London, Routledge and Kegan Paul, 1953.

73 —— *The construction of reality in the child*, London, *Ibid*, 1954.

74 Pincus, L and Dare, C *Secrets in the Family*, London, Faber and Faber, 1978.

75 Ragg, N M *People not Cases: A Philosophical Approach to Social Work*, London, Routledge and Kegan Paul, 1977.

76 Rapaport, R N *Community as Doctor*, London, Tavistock, 1960.

77 Rosen, G 'Madness in society', in *The Historical Sociology of Mental Illness*, London, Routledge and Kegan Paul, 1968.

78 Rutter, M 'Classification and Categorisation in Child Psychiatry', *Journal of Child Psychology and Psychiatry*, 6, 71–83, 1965.

79 —— *Maternal Deprivation Reassessed*, Harmondsworth, Penguin, 1972.

80 —— *Changing Youth in a Changing Society*, London, Nuffield Provincial Hospitals Trust, 1979.

81 —— *Helping Troubled Children*, Harmondsworth, Penguin, 1975.

82 —— 'Speech delay', in 85, 1977.

83 Rutter, M L, Cox, A, Tupling, C, Berger, M and Yule, W 'Attainment and Adjustment in Two Geographical Areas. I: The Prevalence of Psychiatric Disorder, *Brit. J. Psychiat.*, 126, 493–509, 1975.

84 Rutter, M, Graham, P, Chadwick, O and Yule, W 'Adolescent Turmoil: Fact or Fiction?', *Journal of Child Psychology and Psychiatry*, 17, 35–56, 1976.

85 Rutter, M and Hersov, L *Child Psychiatry: Modern Approaches*, Oxford, Blackwell, 1977.

86 Rutter, M and Madge, N *Cycles of Disadvantage*, London, Heinemann, 1977.

87 Rutter, M 'Individual Differences', in 85, 1977.

88 Rutter, M, Shaffer, D and Shepherd, M *A Multi-Axial Classification of Child Psychiatric Disorders*, Geneva, World Health Organisation, 1975.

89 Rutter, M, Shaffer, D and Sturge, C *A Guide to a Multi-Axial Classification Scheme for Psychiatric Disorders in Childhood and Adolescence*, London, Institute of Psychiatry, 1975.

90 Rutter, M, Tizard, J and Whitmore, K *Education, Health and Behaviour*, London, Longman, 1970.

91 Schopler, E and Reichler, R J 'Developmental Therapy by Parents with their own Autistic Child', in Rutter, M (Ed), *Infantile Autism: Concepts, Characteristics and Treatment*, London, Churchill Livingstone, 1971.

92 Shaffer, D 'Suicide in Childhood and Early Adolescence', *Journal of Child Psychology and Psychiatry*, 15, 275–292, 1974.

93 Shaffer, D 'Drug treatment', in 85, 1977.

94 Shaffer, D 'Enuresis', in 85, 1977.

95 Skynner, A C R *One Flesh: Separate Persons. Principles of Family and Marital Psychotherapy*, London, Constable, 1976.

96 Stafford-Clark, D *What Freud Really Said*, Harmondsworth, Penguin, 1969.

97 Steinberg, D 'Psychotic Disorders in Adolescence', in 85, 1977.

98 —— 'The Use of Lithium Carbonate in Adolescence', *Journal of Child Psychology and Psychiatry*, 21, 263–271, 1980.

99 —— 'Two Years' Referrals to a Regional Adolescent Unit', *Social Science and Medicine* (in press), 1981.

100 —— 'The Clinical Psychiatry of Adolescence', Chichester, John Wiley (in preparation).

101 Steinberg, D, Merry, J and Collins, S 'The Introduction

of Small Group Work to an Adolescent Unit', *Journal of Adolescence*, 1, 331–44, 1978.

102 Taylor, D C 'Some psychiatric aspects of epilepsy', in *Current Problems in Neuropsychiatry*, R. N. Hetherington (Ed), Ashford, Kent, Headley Brothers, 1969.

103 Thompson, J W '"Burnout" in group home houseparents', *American Journal of Psychiatry*, 137, 6, 710–714, 1980.

104 Tizard, B *Adoption: A Second Chance*, London, Open Books, 1977.

105 Tizard, J. The Upbringing of Other People's Children: Implications of Research and for Research, *Journal of Child Psychology and Psychiatry*, 15, 161–173, 1974.

106 Tyrer, P and Steinberg, D *Models for Mental Disorder*, (in preparation).

107 Warren, W 'Child Psychiatry and the Maudsley Hospital: An Historical Survey', in *Institute of Psychiatry 1924–1974*, London, Institute of Psychiatry, 1975.

108 Whitmore, K 'The Contribution of Child Guidance to the Community', Paper given at the 30th Child Guidance Inter-Clinic Conference, March 1974.

109 Wing, L (Ed) *Early Childhood Autism: Clinical, Educational and Social Aspects*, Oxford, Pergamon, 1976.

110 Wing, L 'Childhood Autism and Social Class: A Question of Selection?' *British Journal of Psychiatry*, 137, 410–417, 1980.

111 Winnicott, D W *The Maturational Processes and the Facilitating Environment*, London, The Hogarth Press, 1972.

112 —— *Playing and Reality*, Harmondsworth, Penguin, 1974.

113 —— 'Contemporary Concepts of Adolescent Development and their Implications for Higher Education', in 112, 1974.

114 Wolkind, S and Rutter, M 'Children who have been "In Care" – an Epidemiological Study', *Journal of Child Psychology and Psychiatry*, 14, 97–105, 1973.

115 Wolkind, S and Renton, G 'Psychiatric Disorders in Children in Long-term Residential Care: A Follow-up Study', *British Journal of Psychiatry*, 135, 129–135, 1979.

116   World Health Organisation, *The International Pilot Study of Schizophrenia*, vol. 1, WHO, Geneva, 1973.

117   Wolff, S 'Non-delinquent Disturbances of Conduct', in 85, 1977.

118   Wyss, D *Depth Psychology: A Critical History*, London, George Allen and Unwin, 1966.

119   Yule, W, Berger, M and Howlin, P 'Language Deficit and Behaviour Modification', in O'Connor, N (Ed) *Language, Cognition Defect and Retardation*, London, Butterworths, 1975.

120   Yule, W 'Behavioural approaches', in 85, 1977.

Index

UNDERSTANDING AGEING

MELISSA HARDIE

Until this century, the number of people who lived to be very old was proportionately insignificant and those who did survive were usually well cared for in the family. Today the situation is very different – the general expectation of life is much longer, the proportion of the population in the elderly bracket is growing steadily and most of the elderly can lead, and want to lead, independent and active lives.

This is a book of practical advice covering every aspect of life and the problems and choices which the elderly, or their relatives, may face, for example, where to live, adaptations in the home, the importance of health, exercise, sleep and food, opportunities for work. Throughout there are full details on the organised help available and how the bodies concerned may be contacted.

Melissa Hardie includes advice both for the elderly living alone and for those who have an elderly member of the family living with them. The aim throughout is to demonstrate that old age is a precious period in our lives to be planned for and lived to the full in the same way as any other stage.

Melissa Hardie, BA, SRN, is Research Associate at the Nursing Research Unit, Edinburgh University.

TEACH YOURSELF BOOKS

CHILDREN WITH HANDICAPS

LORNA SELFE AND LYNN STOW

This wide-ranging survey considers every aspect of children's handicaps – physical, sensory and intellectual, specific learning difficulties, language problems, social disadvantages and emotional maladjustment – giving practical advice oriented towards remedial help. The emphasis throughout is on positive achievement. Recent trends in educational practice and legislation are examined, and the findings of the Warnock Report discussed. Coming to terms with parenting a handicapped child and a comprehensive list of helping organisations are also included.

Teachers, social workers and medical staff will find this book invaluable and parents of handicapped children will appreciate its positive approach and practical advice.

Lorna Selfe is an educational psychologist who works and researches in the field of children's handicaps. Lynn Stow currently lectures and researches in educational psychology and has worked with children with learning difficulties.

TEACH YOURSELF BOOKS

DRUGS IN PERSPECTIVE

MARTIN A. PLANT

A lucid and non-alarmist approach to the often emotive subject of mind-altering drugs, reflecting current research and thinking and placing all drugs, whether 'social', 'illicit', or 'prescribed' in their proper perspective.

Tobacco and alcohol, tranquillisers and sleeping pills, illicit drugs – the effects, legal status and patterns of use of each are discussed, and the author identifies the social and age groups at risk in each case. He considers the underlying causes of the increase in drug consumption in the West in recent years and critically appraises treatment of drug problems.

This is a book for anyone interested in the subject of drug consumption and its social effects, and will be particularly helpful to those whose work involves contact with drug problems.

TEACH YOURSELF BOOKS

UNDERSTANDING DYSLEXIA

T. R. MILES

One of the most important things for a dyslexic child is that his difficulties should be understood. In the past many such children have been considered stupid or lazy when in fact they were neither.

It is now widely recognised that there may be some kind of constitutionally caused limitation, due neither to lack of intelligence nor to emotional or social difficulties, as a result of which some people are late in learning to read, find spelling very hard, and have all kinds of difficulties in 'getting things in the right order'.

Professor Miles here describes how dyslexic children can be recognised and how provision can be made, both at school and in the home, for helping them.

This book is essential reading for parents and for all those, such as doctors, teachers and social workers, who are involved with dyslexic children in their professional lives.

TEACH YOURSELF BOOKS

PSYCHOLOGY FOR TODAY

ED. BILL GILLHAM

This introductory text by past and present members of Nottingham University's Department of Psychology surveys what has been described as 'the most important human science'. Each author is an expert on the subject he discusses and the book as a whole reflects, in summary, current thinking on all the major areas of psychology studied at universities and polytechnics.

The 'non-technical' language makes this book suitable for a wide readership and it will be particularly useful in sixth forms as an advanced course and at first-year undergraduate level. Each chapter is intended as an introduction to its subject and contains a comprehensive list of references for further reading.

A lively and wide-ranging collaboration, the book goes a long way towards meeting what its editor considers the greatest challenge to psychology today – 'communicating its methods and findings to people at large'.

TEACH YOURSELF BOOKS